THE DECAF DIET

Warning and Disclaimer

The ideas, concepts, and opinions expressed in this book are intended to be helpful and informative on the subject addressed. This book is not intended as a substitute for medical advice from a healthcare professional. The author, editors, and publisher assume no responsibility for any outcome of applying the ideas and concepts in this book in a program of self-care or under the care of a qualified healthcare professional. Exercise programs may cause injuries, and you should receive full medical clearance from a licensed physician before beginning any exercise program. If you have questions about any of the recommendations in this book, you should consult a qualified healthcare professional.

THE DECAF DIET

IS CAFFEINE MAKING YOU FAT?

EUGENE WELLS

CONTENTS

Why, this Satan's drink is so delicious, that it would be a pity to let the infidels have exclusive use of it. We shall fool Satan by baptizing it and making it a truly Christian beverage.

-Pope Clement VIII, referring to coffee[1]

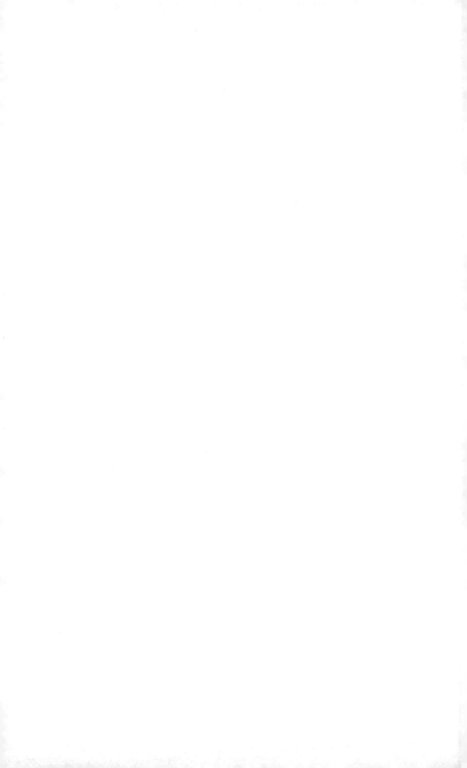

PREFACE

Why I Wrote This Book

Up until a certain point in my life, I was able to eat whatever I wanted in whatever quantity I wanted, while remaining lean. I would eat, and eat, and eat, but my flat stomach remained. Among other things, I would eat pints of ice cream as snacks before bed, often with peanut butter mixed into them. Yes, I really took advantage of my inability to gain weight. Thoughts of overeating and weight gain never even crossed my mind. I loved being able to eat so much without gaining weight.

As you can guess, I got my comeuppance. My ability to stay lean suddenly changed when I was in my mid-twenties, and fat started to accumulate rapidly around my mid-section. I ignored it at first, but after putting on 35 pounds in six months, I knew I had to address my sudden weight gain. The weight I had put on in this short span of time was especially unsightly on my body given my narrow frame. I am tall, but very lanky, so when my belly appeared, I not only looked fat, I looked ridiculous. My belly stood out and overshadowed the rest of my body, and I was not happy with my appearance.

So I began to investigate the origins of my weight gain and possible ways to drop the weight. I wondered if something had changed in my diet or if perhaps my "fast metabolism" had finally abandoned me. Maybe I wasn't working out enough. I tried different approaches to lose the weight but I could not get it to come off and stay off, so I began to believe that my metabolism had in fact slowed down. In trying to lose the weight, I embarked on various diets and exercise regimens, most of which were helpful at first, but whatever weight I lost on these programs I soon gained back.

Finally, I reexamined what had changed in my life at the precise point when I began to gain weight. The only significant difference was the addition of moderate amounts of caffeine to my diet. All of the weight gain had occurred immediately after I began to consume caffeine on a daily basis. The point at which I began to drink upwards of four cups of green and black tea a day coincided exactly with the beginning of my weight gain.

At first I thought this was just a coincidence. The two should not be related, after all, the media and fitness experts tell us that caffeine makes us lose weight, not put it on. With the amounts of green tea I was drinking, I should have been leaner than ever! Not so. I began investigating the effects of caffeine on weight gain, and my findings were surprising, to say the least. I also discovered that I was by far not the only person to associate caffeine consumption with weight gain.

This book is the culmination of my research efforts, and I believe its contents will prove helpful to the confused and frustrated dieter, as it would have been very helpful to me at an earlier point in my own life. Together, we will explore the causes of and solutions to weight gain, as I describe the connections between caffeine consumption and the stubborn accumulation of body fat. I hope that with the strategies contained in the following chapters, we can all become leaner, healthier individuals. If it is any enticement, the strategies worked for me, I have my flat stomach back, and I have not gotten any younger.

In writing this book, I made myself a guinea pig both to make sure that caffeine was fattening for me, and to test out different ways of reducing, eliminating, and manipulating caffeine intake to determine which methods were the most effective for weight loss. I put myself through ten deliberate cycles of getting on and off caffeine so that I would have a familiar, personal understanding of its effects and the difficulties in quitting, in order to share with you the best of what I discovered.

Caffeine and Diet

The dietary advice landscape is a confusing one. There are a large number of weight loss diets that promise results through as large a number of different strategies. When we are trying to lose weight or maintain a lean weight, we generally try some diets, pick the ones we like and try to stay on them long enough to reach our weight loss goals. Our diets usually don't last long, however, and we often quit in frustration. The caffeinated beverage landscape, in comparison, is not so confusing or frustrating. There is a large variety of caffeinated beverages, with many different flavors, but this landscape is not difficult to navigate. We try a few caffeinated beverages, pick the ones we like, and typically drink these beverages for life. Finding a diet that keeps us lean and that we can keep for life is far more difficult.

What is the relationship between caffeine intake and weight loss? How does caffeine fit into a weight loss diet, and does it fit at all? Does caffeine encourage weight loss or does it hinder weight loss? The answers are often unclear. Some health experts allow coffee and tea on a weight loss diet, so long as these beverages are taken without large amounts of cream and sugar. Other health experts forbid caffeinated beverages entirely, warning that caffeine contributes to weight gain all by itself. Does it?

It does, and I'll explain how. In fact it is not much of a stretch to state that caffeine use and the particular ways in which we take caffeine are some of the main causes of weight gain and obesity in modern society. Armed with a wealth of new research, we can now reach the conclusion that caffeine is fattening with confidence. Regular caffeine consumption encourages overeating, making weight loss and lasting leanness very difficult to achieve.

That being said, I will not ask you to give up your favorite caffeinated foods and beverages completely, and perhaps not at all, depending on your particular health and weight loss goals. What I will do, is explain how you can reduce or modify your caffeine intake to maximize your body's leanness and minimize caffeine's fattening effects. Insofar as an individual's body weight is concerned, the phrase, "drink responsibly" applies to caffeine.

I would like to raise awareness of caffeine's role in weight gain and to contribute meaningfully to the nutritional discourse. I am not a hater of happiness, nor am I a hater of caffeine, and I would rather the evidence proved that caffeine was an elixir of health. Unfortunately, that is not the case, especially in the area of weight gain, and there is a significant amount of evidence that caffeine causes overeating and slows metabolism through a number of biological mechanisms.

Caffeine is our favorite stimulant, enthralling us with its effects, and as a species we have become nothing more than slaves to this drug. The plants that originally produced it as a pesticide now have such sway over us as their caretakers to ensure their indefinite survival on this planet. Holding center stage in our society, caffeine is unlike other drugs in that its consumption is completely socially acceptable. Moreover, society even expects us to use this drug in order to be productive individuals.

Caffeine backs us into a corner wherever we go. It is unavoidable, greeting us in its many incarnations, including coffee, tea, soda, energy drinks, chocolate, and prescription and non-prescription drugs. If we don't have our morning cup of coffee before we leave for work, then we have many opportunities to get our caffeine fix on the way to work at one of many coffeehouses and grocery stores. Most offices provide their employees with complimentary coffee and tea, and when that is not the case, the cafeteria, vending machine, or convenience store is never far.

We have a natural obsession with caffeine. Being a stimulant, caffeine often makes us feel good, apparently gives us the energy we need to continue working and achieving, and it's legal! It is no wonder that we reserve a special place in our lives for this drug, often offering one of its carrier beverages to guests and sharing caffeinated beverages with close friends and loved ones. But no matter how much we love and depend on a mainstay of our modern human diet, it is important to question the health implications of our food staples, especially when the staple in question is a drug.

The effects of caffeine on the human body are numerous and complicated. For purposes of this book, I am interested only in the effects of caffeine on fat gain and fat loss in the human body. Considering the obesity epidemic and the myriad health complications that come with obesity and weight gain in general, examining the effects of caffeine in this realm is both worthy and timely. Restricting myself to this particular area still leaves me with an almost endless supply of interesting issues to talk about. This book's purpose is to address those individuals who are having trouble losing weight while regularly consuming caffeine, so just about everyone in the United States, and perhaps the world.

Dietary caffeine contributes to fat gain while at the same time hindering fat loss. I describe how caffeine does so in detail in the following chapters. Since it will be a while before we get there, I will give you my recommendations here so that you may have them from the start. First, we must strive to reduce our caffeine consumption, but it is not necessary to eliminate caffeine altogether. Second, we must choose better sources of caffeine in our diets and better ways of consuming caffeine that take into account its fattening effects. Third, when we do consume caffeine, we must make some dietary and lifestyle adjustments in order to blunt caffeine's fattening effects.

A Note on References

Many publishers insist that in writing a book for the general public, footnotes and endnotes should be stripped from the main text as so much confusing clutter. I disagree with this notion and I would feel uncomfortable with simply listing my sources for each of my chapters at the end of this book, instead of letting you know exactly which sources I am using to support specific propositions. I think it is best for you to have a clear path from the text to the sources that I used, so that you can easily check my work. I often cite multiple sources for the same propositions, just in case you have difficulty finding some of the sources I relied on. I recommend all the books that I have cited in my references, as I found them all to be very interesting. As for the scholarly articles, I recommend those as well if you enjoy reading them.

A Note on Organization

I'd like to give you a quick roadmap of where I'm going before we start. That way you can have a view of the forest before we begin to walk among the trees. In the first chapter, Paradigms, I will establish a framework for thinking about caffeine's effects on overeating and metabolism, and this framework will stay with us for the remainder of the book. In Chapter 2, Meet Caffeine, we will become better acquainted with caffeine and its carrier beverages and foods. In chapters 3-6, we will examine caffeine's fattening properties in depth, and I will strive to organize some of the overlapping issues in as logical a manner as I can.

In Chapter 7, The Decaf Plan, I will describe how to reduce or eliminate your caffeine consumption painlessly, in order to better achieve your weight loss goals. In Chapter 8, Optimal Caffeine Use, I will describe how to use caffeine properly, so its fattening effects are reduced as much as possible. Chapter 8 may be the most important chapter in the book because I recognize that a complete elimination of caffeine or even a reduction may be impractical or undesirable for many people. Finally, in Chapter 9, Lasting Leanness, I try to tie all of the previous chapters together into a mind-blowing and life-altering conclusion. That's a bit much to go for, but I promise to make it interesting and we'll see what happens.

You will find a number of recommendations scattered throughout this book, but don't worry about taking notes because I will recap the most important recommendations in chapters 7 and 8. In addition, I have included a summary paragraph at the conclusion of each of chapters 1-8, going over the most important points of each of these chapters, for your quick reference.

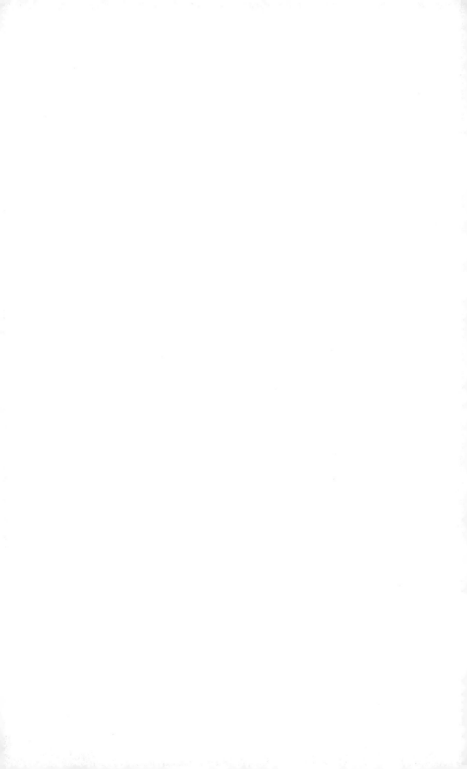

CHAPTER 1
PARADIGMS

If you write in a category, you write knowing there's a framework, there are reader expectations.

-Nora Roberts

Something happened in the United States in the early 1980s. Obesity had already been on the rise in the United States and throughout the world, but in the early 1980s, obesity rates began to accelerate as never before. Since that time, we have been getting fatter at an alarming rate, and the upward trend in obesity rates does not show any signs of slowing. Besides the aesthetic frustrations that come with obesity, there are also countless health problems that threaten not only to cost billions of dollars to treat, but also to decrease our collective and individual enjoyment of life.

Leading diabetes and obesity researchers are racing against the clock, trying to figure out how to stop the rapidly progressing obesity epidemic. The researchers know what causes obesity, and how to create weight loss in controlled environments. What remains unclear, however, is the best way to treat obesity in real life, and on a grand scale. In this chapter we will explore the basic weight loss concepts that researchers agree upon. We will also consider why some diets succeed while others fail, and I will provide you with a weight loss framework in which to view the rest of the information in this book.

Energy Balance

Are you wondering about the Nora Roberts quote? I include it because I understand that I am writing in the diet genre, a genre that is admittedly bloated itself. You are probably wondering if this is another low carbohydrate diet, or another low fat diet, as these are currently the dominant dietary frameworks. *The Decaf Diet* is neither of these. Instead of focusing on a particular food list of allowed or disallowed foods, I focus only on the role that caffeine plays in overeating, and how to overcome caffeine's fattening effects.

My framework is that of overeating being the cause both of weight gain and the diseases that are associated with weight gain. I view caffeine consumption in terms of its effects on overeating, and it is from that vantage point that I make the recommendations in this book. Before moving on to the particulars of caffeine's impact on our waistlines, let's discuss some dietary frameworks, become familiar with the basics of these frameworks, and in this way begin our discussion of caffeine with a background understanding of what it takes to lose weight and keep it off.

The only valid, inclusive framework with which to view weight gain and weight loss is that of energy balance. The two energy balance variables that control weight gain and weight loss are energy intake and energy expenditure. Energy intake is food intake, and energy expenditure is the body's use of food energy throughout the day. Energy expenditure includes the body's burning of energy both while at rest and while engaged in physical activity. When energy intake exceeds energy expenditure for a given period of time, we enter positive energy balance, and weight gain occurs. When energy expenditure exceeds energy intake for a given period of time, we enter negative energy balance, and weight loss occurs. Medical professionals and obesity researchers agree that energy balance determines whether we gain weight or lose it, and that obesity can be treated *only* by reducing energy intake (eating less) or increasing energy expenditure (exercising more).

In the context of diet, energy is often measured in calories. A calorie is a unit of energy that we use to measure the energy we receive from food and that we expend in our daily activities. One calorie is the amount of energy necessary to increase the temperature of one liter of water by one degree centigrade, at sea level. By decreasing food intake enough, or by increasing physical activity enough, an individual can reach the point of negative calorie balance (negative energy balance), where energy intake is less than energy expenditure in a given period of time. Once our hypothetical dieter reaches and maintains negative calorie balance for a long enough period of time, he will lose weight. Negative calorie balance can be described as undereating, and positive energy balance can be described as overeating.

There are several ways to achieve negative calorie balance. The dieter can decrease calorie intake while keeping calories burned constant; or increase calories burned while keeping calorie intake constant; or decrease calorie intake and increase calories burned simultaneously. Those are the only "weighs" to do it. Sorry about that, I am a sucker for bad puns. But that is the formula for weight loss. The formula is simple enough, but sustaining negative calorie balance is more difficult in practice than it is on paper. Most dieters fail to lose weight, and when they do succeed they often find themselves gaining back all of the weight they lost.

While researchers and diet experts agree that decreasing food intake and increasing physical activity are the keys to weight loss, they disagree on which of these two strategies should receive the most attention from dieters seeking lasting weight loss. Some researchers contend that adding

3

regular exercise to our lives is the answer. Others contend that any weight loss effort can succeed only through diet, because our diet is the most modifiable part of the energy balance equation, whereas modern sedentary life makes regular exercise impractical.

Yet other researchers point to the increase in food intake and simultaneous decrease in physical activity that took place in the last century and argue that any effective weight loss plan must both decrease food intake and increase physical activity. All of these approaches have value, and the viability of each approach depends on the circumstances of individual dieters. Some have time for exercise, others do not. For those who can not exercise and who must sit at work to earn a living, a greater burden necessarily falls on the food intake half of the calorie equation.

A number of different factors are responsible for the common inability to achieve negative calorie balance and sustain it. First, we can look at North American culture, with its emphasis on large portion sizes and calorie-dense eating at fast food restaurants. North American culture is rapidly spreading throughout the world, and the fast food culture is no longer a local phenomenon. Second, we can try to explain why we overeat from a biological perspective. This explanation focuses on how our food choices, hormones, and environments affect our feelings of satiety (feelings of being full) and our desire to overeat.

Our caffeine consumption makes negative calorie balance very difficult to achieve and maintain. As I will explain in detail in the upcoming chapters, caffeine contributes significantly to overeating in a number of different ways. Since I do not expect to change the cultural aspects of American life that contribute to overeating through this book, I will focus on how to remove the biological impediments to achieving negative calorie balance, and the biological impediments to staying out of positive calorie balance. In other words, the recommendations in this book will help you reduce your food intake and achieve negative calorie balance with little effort, simply by modifying your caffeine intake.

Hormonal Balance

Hormonal factors and other non-energy balance variables are only relevant to the weight loss discussion when they affect energy balance by affecting food intake, energy expenditure, or both. There are a great many different weight loss diets. Some focus on calories, others focus on macronutrient ratios (the proportions of dietary fat, protein, and carbohydrate), and yet others focus on hormonal balance. All of these factors – calories, macronutrient ratios, and hormonal balance – are interrelated such that they are inseparable.

Why are there so many diets? I think it is in part because people are always searching for causal relationships to explain the physical world, and there are a great many valid causal relationships that exist, some that are known and others that remain undiscovered. However, it often happens that hormonal balance or macronutrient balance are blamed out of context. Hormonal balance and macronutrient balance are relevant only to the extent that they have an impact on the body's overall energy balance. Hormones can not make you fat, unless they can increase your food intake and/or decrease your energy expenditure significantly enough to create a positive energy balance.

Diet writers sometimes observe two phenomena that present themselves simultaneously, and in trying to establish a causal link between the two, forget about energy balance completely. Even if energy balance were not the most important aspect of changing one's body fat levels, which it is, just because two events occur simultaneously, it does not necessarily follow that one causes the other. On the contrary, both phenomena may have one common explanatory cause, or they may have two or more distinct explanatory causes.

To be slightly less abstract, let's say we are talking about obesity and high levels of hormone X and a high intake of macronutrient Y, which present themselves simultaneously most of the time. The way people usually react to this scenario is by trying to find ways that explain how high levels of hormone X and a high intake of macronutrient Y cause obesity, or how obesity causes high levels of hormone X. Where we sometimes go wrong is in forgetting that another distinct cause, such as overeating (positive energy balance), may be responsible for obesity and high levels of hormone X and a high intake of macronutrient Y. If we begin to believe that overeating is the initial cause of both obesity and high levels of hormone X and a high intake of macronutrient Y, the next point of error is to forget that obesity, hormone X, and a high intake of macronutrient Y, once present, may themselves contribute to overeating, their initial common cause, leading to a self-perpetuating cycle.

In our hypothetical scenario, overeating leads to obesity, high levels of hormone X, and a high intake of macronutrient Y. Hormone X and a high intake of macronutrient Y in turn increase our overeating behavior by making us have food cravings for specific foods. Overeating may also cause high levels of hormone Z, which rather than creating cravings, decreases our ability to feel full, and contributes to overeating indirectly. What am I trying to say with this alphabet soup? My point is that what and how much we eat affect our hormones, and our hormones also affect what and how much we eat. To blame hormones alone, or to blame macronutrients alone, is to paint an incomplete

6

picture, and biology does not allow for this kind of oversimplification.

This notion of interrelationships will crystallize as we continue our discussion. For now, let's continue by deconstructing popular notions about metabolism and the most popular dietary frameworks, with an aim at understanding the difference between dietary success and failure. We will then explore how caffeine helps to put most weight loss efforts in the failure category.

Metabolism

Metabolism is one of the favorite buzzwords of the diet and fitness communities. I'll admit it, I like it too. It's a sexy term. In the mainstream parlance metabolism refers to an individual's rate of fat-burning while at rest, as distinguished from that individual's rate of fat-burning while engaged in physical activity. Metabolism refers to the energy expenditure that takes place while we are lounging about, reading the paper, watching television, and so forth. We are all told that as we get older, our bodies begin to slow down and burn calories at a slower rate, thus making it more and more difficult to stay lean. Many people even have their own theories about the precise age at which our metabolisms slow down, the point from which "it's all downhill."

A friend of mine insists that 25 is the magical age when the body begins to shut down and everything starts to break and shift into low gear. Of course, it is impossible to pinpoint a specific age that can be generalized among all people, but most of us come to accept that a slowing metabolism is an inevitable part of getting older, as is the fat gain that invariably accompanies aging. But to what extent can we really blame our metabolisms for making us gain weight? Do those of us who are prone to weight gain have slow metabolisms when compared to those of us who stay lean?

Before we answer this question, let's explore the origins of the idea that a slow metabolism causes weight gain. With vehemence and vitriol, many contemporary diet writers proclaim that calories don't matter. Why is "calories don't matter" the clarion call of some diet promoters, most notably promoters of the low carbohydrate diet, and to some extent of the low fat, whole foods, and vegan diets? This anti-calorie propaganda originated when some dieters began to claim that they could not lose weight no matter how little they ate or how much they exercised. These problem dieters were supposedly unable to lose weight while on low calorie diets, but then eventually were successful on a low carbohydrate or other diet that promises hormonal benefits that are allegedly more important than calorie balance. Is there in fact such a dieter to whom the energy balance equation does not apply? As you can suspect from my tone, the answer is no.

There is a popular mainstream belief that some individuals can gain weight or survive with almost no food, and that obese individuals eat no more, or even less, than lean individuals. Due to the absence of an accurate way to measure an individual's energy expenditure before the 1980s, this belief has prevailed for a long time, and is still common today.[2] Its origin can be traced back to the first dieters who showed up at the doorsteps of doctors and researchers, claiming that they eat very little, and yet can not lose weight or even continue to gain weight. These dieters maintained that they ate almost nothing, exercised, and their weight still would not budge. So the doctors and researchers studied these dieters, and in the absence of an accurate way to measure how much the dieters ate and how much energy they expended during the day, the doctors and researchers were forced to rely on the dieters' own reports of their daily food intake and activity levels. The result is that much obesity research was done by researchers relying on the self-reported food intakes of dieters.

A reliance on the self-reporting of food intake led to the proliferation of the "calories don't count" phenomenon that we still see today, lending support to the notion that a slow metabolism causes weight gain. Self-reporting is notoriously inaccurate and unreliable, but there is so much of this erroneous data that many diet writers have relied on and continue to rely on self-reported accounts of food intake.[3] The researchers who have relied on this inaccurate data have concluded that the overweight and obese eat less than the lean, that the amount of food eaten has no relation to body weight, and therefore that overeating has nothing to do with the obesity epidemic.[4]

The following quote from a leading obesity researcher sums it up nicely: "[t]he unlikely possibility that the laws of thermodynamics need reconsideration or that humans can generate energy by photosynthesis can probably be discounted."[5] This quote is made funnier by the fact that some individuals claim they can survive by feeding on sunlight, in the absence of food. Putting these notions to rest once and for all, the doubly labeled water method, which was perfected for use in humans in the early 1980s, allows researchers to accurately measure an individual's energy expenditure.

Researchers employ the doubly labeled water method by administering water to subjects in which the hydrogen and oxygen have been replaced by less common isotopes of these elements (this water is said to be traced, or labeled). The researchers are then able to accurately determine the subjects' metabolic rates by taking saliva, blood, and urine samples, measuring the rate at which subjects eliminate the labeled water.

This measurement technique finally enabled researchers to examine the hypothesis that overweight individuals eat less than lean individuals and yet remain overweight. Unsurprisingly, this hypothesis was found not to hold water. Studies using the doubly labeled water method described above have highlighted the inaccuracy of self-reported food logs, and have demonstrated that the inaccuracy of self-reported food intake increases with an individual's weight.[6] Dieters frequently underreport their daily food intakes, even when researchers thoroughly train these dieters to accurately keep food logs.[7] Instead of recording their actual food intakes, dieters tend to record food intakes that are much lower, and the heavier a dieter is, the worse is his degree of underreporting.

In one study that examined the disparity between self-reported intakes and actual intakes as measured by the doubly labeled water method, the participants underestimated their food intakes by an average of more than 1000 calories per day.[8] In some cases the participants, whom researchers thoroughly instructed on how to take accurate records, were self-reporting only half of their actual food intakes! Overweight and obese individuals do in fact have higher food intakes than lean individuals, and at this point in our discussion this should be no surprise.[9] A number of studies have shown that the degree of underreporting is usually less severe than 50%, and ranges from 20-40% less than actual energy intake, which is still a considerable level of underreporting.[10]

What are some causes of the underreporting phenomenon? One of the main causes is that most of us tend to fill out food logs in ways that show us in a favorable light, both to portray a positive image to others and to ourselves.[11] Whether we do this consciously or subconsciously, inaccurate self-reporting can be viewed as a self-protective technique, but it is disadvantageous when weight loss is our ultimate goal. Another significant cause of underreporting is the mislabeling of foods. The textbook weight of some foods (found in calorie references for dieters) is often far below the weight of these foods in real life, and some foods that are marketed as "diet" foods often contain many more calories than their labels state.[12] This is true mostly for local and regional "diet" foods, as nationally promoted "diet" foods are more careful with their labeling.

Keeping accurate food logs and counting calories is difficult to do accurately outside of the laboratory, so it has led to the belief that calories are not important. It's not that calories don't count, it's that we can't and don't have the time or energy to count calories. Diets work best when they don't require their participants to count calories, but create satiety, which results in an automatic down-regulation of food intake. Moreover, feelings of hunger and satiety are not necessarily functions of calorie intake. The ideal way to lose weight is to reduce food cravings so that food intake automatically decreases, and simultaneously increase the body's metabolic rate.

As we'll soon see, manipulating our caffeine intakes can have a profound impact on our feelings of satiety, and a significant impact on our resting energy expenditure. The bottom line is that self-recorded food logs are not accurate, and now that we have accurate and reliable methods for measuring energy intake and energy expenditure, we can return to the meaningful framework of energy balance and seek our weight loss goals with the aid of logic and objectivity.

Most of us who gain weight and find it difficult to lose do not suffer from a "slow metabolism." The doubly labeled water method finally enabled researchers to examine the hypothesis that fat gain is the result of having a slow metabolism, and studies using this method do not support the old and popular notion that weight gain and obesity are caused by a slow metabolism.[13] These studies did not find that overweight people have slow metabolisms.

On the contrary, the research demonstrates that many overweight and obese individuals have metabolic rates faster than those of lean individuals.[14] Overweight and obese individuals actually have a greater average energy expenditure than lean individuals, due to the increase in energy-consuming muscle mass that comes with weight gain and the increased energy demand on the body to support extra weight. Furthermore, research also does not support the popular notion that undereating and low calorie diets slow an individual's metabolism, making weight loss difficult or impossible.[15]

The notion of a "slow metabolism" as the cause of weight gain is appealing but dangerous. Believing the slow metabolism hype lets us shift the responsibility for our weight gain away from ourselves and onto our supposedly malfunctioning bodies. It leads to thinking that "I am not overweight because of factors that I can control, such as my food intake and level of physical activity, but because of my treacherous metabolism."

The danger in this kind of thinking, aside from its falsity, is that we give up control of our weight problems to the somewhat abstract notion of metabolism, and as a result we can feel justified in inaction. If our metabolisms are "slow," we are powerless in the struggle to lose weight, so why try? The "slow metabolism" idea breeds resignation and inaction, and in many cases is an excuse to avoid changing our eating and exercise habits.

Aside from the finding that a slow metabolism is not the cause of weight gain, there is another point you should take away from the above studies. That is the finding that your rate of fat burning while at rest is affected most significantly by the amount of fat-free mass in your body, so maintaining high levels of muscle mass will give you some metabolic advantage, however small.[16]

While a slow metabolism does not make us fat, it may still be desirable to aim for the slight metabolic boost that increased muscle mass provides, if we can experience this boost in conjunction with a reduced food intake. That being said, your rate of fat-burning at rest is not as important for maintaining leanness as is your level of physical activity.[17] An individual's rate of fat burning while the body is at rest has very little impact on that individual's propensity to gain weight. Instead, the most important variable that affects an individual's total energy expenditure is the amount of physical activity that individual performs. Regular exercise makes it more likely that the weight loss you experience will be permanent, and the common post-diet weight regain will not occur.[18]

While it is rare for an individual to be suffering from a slow metabolism, it does happen in certain cases, for example, it may occur in individuals who were previously treated for an overactive thyroid and who are currently on certain medications.[19] In cases like this, it is not unusual for the individual metabolic rate to be approximately 25% below average.

Although having a slow metabolism like this is rare, I want to cover all of the bases so I will focus on increasing your resting metabolic rate as well as your level of physical activity, so we can address the energy expenditure part of the equation from all the angles. While the metabolic boost you receive from carrying some extra muscle is modest, every little bit counts, and we'll discuss how to increase and maintain your muscle mass in several of the upcoming chapters.

As you'll soon see, caffeine consumption has a direct effect on the amount of muscle mass you carry (it's not a positive one).

The Thermic Effect

Since we are talking about metabolism and energy expenditure, this is as good a time as any to introduce the thermic effect of food. The thermic effect of food is the amount of energy that the body must expend in digesting food to break it down into substances that it can use for growth, repair, maintenance, and energy. The three macronutrients, carbohydrates, fat, and protein, have different thermic effects. Each of these macronutrients takes a different amount of energy to digest. The thermic effect of protein is approximately 20-35% of ingested calories; the thermic effect of carbohydrates is approximately 15-25% of ingested calories; and the thermic effect of fat is approximately 5-10% of ingested calories.[20]

The practical application of this information is the conclusion that fat is the most efficiently stored macronutrient, followed by carbohydrate, and then protein. By most efficiently stored, I mean that our bodies can get the most energy out of this macronutrient to store as fat, so if weight loss is your concern, you want to avoid foods that the body stores with the greatest efficiency. The overfeeding of protein results in 65-80% of excess energy being stored; overfeeding of carbohydrate results in 75-85% of the excess energy being stored; and overfeeding of fat results in 90-95% of the excess energy being stored. On average, if we ignore the differences among macronutrients, the thermic effect of food is about 10% of the food's calorie content.[21]

Let's illustrate the thermic effect with the following example. If we eat 25 grams of protein, which is 100 calories on paper, our bodies will be able to extract about 65-80 calories of usable energy from this serving of protein. If we eat 25 grams of carbohydrate, which is also 100 calories, our bodies will be able to extract about 75-85 calories of usable energy from this serving of carbohydrate.

If we eat approximately 11 grams of fat, the equivalent of 100 calories, our bodies will be able to extract 90-95 calories of usable energy from this serving of fat. Fat requires the least amount of energy to digest, protein requires the most, and carbohydrate is in the middle. So if our goal is to increase our energy expenditure in digestion, our meals should consist mainly of protein. I mention this for purposes of illustration, and not as a recommendation to adopt a high protein diet.

You probably noticed that 25 grams of protein or carbohydrate both contain 100 calories, but only 11 grams of fat contain 100 calories. This is because fat is a denser source of calories than either protein or carbohydrate, with more than twice as much energy per gram. This is one of the rationales for eliminating or reducing fat consumption for weight loss, as relatively small amounts contain large amounts of calories. This concept brings us to the next section, concerning diets that prefer certain macronutrients over others.

Macronutrient Discrimination

Weight gain is the result of a small or large positive calorie balance that persists over time.[22] In other words, weight gain is the result of overeating relative to your energy expenditure for a period of time. It doesn't matter what macronutrient your extra calories come from, whether it is protein, carbohydrate, or fat, if you are eating more than your body can burn in a given period of time, you will gain weight.

Excess energy is stored as fat, regardless of its source.[23] However, two popular dietary frameworks, those of the low fat and the low carbohydrate diets, often focus their blame on a single macronutrient as being responsible for weight gain to a greater degree than other macronutrients. To some extent, diets that favor certain nutrients over others are on to something, but only when favoring certain macronutrients makes it easier to undereat or to avoid overeating.

Low fat diets discriminate against fat, while low carbohydrate diets discriminate against carbohydrate. Each of these diets claims that it works better than the other, and each claims to bestow on its dieters a wealth of health benefits that the opposing diet does not. And of course, followers of one always threaten followers of the other with various diseases. I believe that these two diets can coexist peacefully, and I hope that one day they shall do so, because they both offer some advantages for dieters. However, some people succeed on one of these diets while failing at the other, so some polarization occurs in the weight loss community around these two opposing dietary ideologies.

What does the research have to say about the relative merits of the low fat and low carbohydrate diets when it comes to lasting weight loss? When the total amount of calories on each diet is held constant, there is no significant variation among the weight loss effects of different diets, including low fat and low carbohydrate regimens.[24] Manipulating the ratios between fat, carbohydrates, and protein has no significant effect on producing weight loss when calories are held constant.

The effectiveness of a 1500 calorie per day weight loss diet will be the same whether the diet is low in fat or low in carbohydrate, as long as you can keep your calorie intake at the prescribed 1500 calories per day. The problem, of course, is staying on the 1500 calories per day for long enough to reach your weight loss goals, and then maintaining that weight loss. Let's move to a closer discussion of the low carbohydrate diet, a diet that often produces success in losing some weight, if not in keeping it off.

Low Carbohydrate Diets

The low carbohydrate diet is in its renaissance, with new incarnations of the low carbohydrate diet cropping up over and over again under different names, and with slight variations among them. Low carbohydrate diets propose that calories are not as important as the source of these calories, and that limiting or eliminating carbohydrates from the diet is the fastest and easiest way to achieve sustainable weight loss.

Low carbohydrate proponents sometimes argue that it is impossible to lose weight or maintain a lean physique while consuming a moderate amount of carbohydrates. The usual rationale behind reducing carbohydrates is that this reduction results in a corresponding reduction in the body's insulin levels, and lower insulin levels hasten fat loss. Insulin control rather than calorie balance, they argue, is the best way to achieve weight loss.

In studies of low carbohydrate diets, however, changes in energy balance, rather than changes in insulin levels, completely account for the weight loss that participants experience.[25] Individuals on low carbohydrate diets spontaneously decrease their calorie intakes, without counting calories. This reduction in energy intake is made possible by increased levels of satiety and therefore reduced hunger on low carbohydrate diets.

17

Calorie reduction, not insulin reduction, is what causes individuals on low carbohydrate diets to lose weight, regardless of whether dieters count their calories. There is a very important lesson here, and that is if we can find ways to increase our levels of satiety, we will begin to eat less automatically. We will explore this concept throughout the rest of this book, as we find ways of altering our caffeine consumption to increase our feelings of fullness, so that we may undereat spontaneously and effortlessly.

When dieters succeed on low carbohydrate regimens, they do so because they have entered negative calorie balance by cutting the amount of carbohydrates in their diets and by cutting their food intakes in general, due to increased feelings of fullness. By eliminating carbohydrates and replacing them with fat and protein, many dieters are able to maintain a lowered calorie intake while feeling full and can thereby undereat relative to their energy expenditures.

However, it remains true that overeating fat or protein does contribute to weight gain. Both fat and protein are stored as fat when they are eaten in excess. Fat and protein are both broken down and either used for energy or for structural purposes, and where those purposes have been fulfilled, these macronutrients are stored in our fat cells, independent of the amount of carbohydrates that is being consumed. Many people gain weight on low carbohydrate diets when they go to extremes and overeat protein and fat, notwithstanding all of the claims that dietary fat and protein will not be stored as fat.

We'll discuss the role of insulin in energy balance in Chapter 4, Caffeine and Insulin, but for now let's address some of the claims made by low carbohydrate advocates that high insulin levels cause weight gain and that low insulin levels cause weight loss. What does the relevant research have to say about the role of insulin levels in weight loss?

18

Low carbohydrate weight loss diets and diets that control insulin levels do not produce any greater weight loss or fat loss than equivalent calorie, high carbohydrate diets.[26] That warrants repeating: insulin, in the absence of overeating and positive calorie balance, does not make a person fat. A comparison of the effects of the Atkins (low carbohydrate), Ornish (very low fat), Weight Watchers (balanced low calorie), and Zone (balanced low calorie) diets for weight loss revealed similar benefits for dieters who were able to stay the course for one year.[27]

Furthermore, as far as their impact on insulin levels, all of these diets, whether they restricted carbohydrates or not, produced a decline in insulin levels along with weight loss. This suggests that high insulin levels are a symptom of overeating, just as weight gain is, rather than the cause or determining factor. Again, we are struck by the truth that energy balance, rather than hormonal balance, is the key to changes in body composition, and hormonal balance is only important for weight loss where it can help us to undereat. (Body composition is the amount of muscle, bone, and fat tissue in the body taken in percentages and evaluated against each other. Our goals for our body compositions in this book are to decrease fat mass and to increase or at least maintain muscle and bone mass.)

The research likewise does not support the popular claim that carbohydrate ingestion makes fat loss impossible by "turning off" fat burning.[28] If this claim were true, then fat loss on low calorie diets that contain moderate levels of carbohydrate would be impossible. On the contrary, all low calorie, moderate, and even high carbohydrate diets produce weight loss when they are carried out in a controlled environment (meaning the researchers are monitoring food intake). Unfortunately, some diet writers go so far as to say that if an individual goes on a low calorie diet and does not restrict carbohydrates, his body will burn muscle for energy, resulting in muscle wasting rather than fat loss. This claim, as you can guess, also is not supported by the studies we have discussed above.

As to the false claim that excess dietary fat is not stored as fat, I can only speculate as to its origins. Fat is incontrovertibly the most efficiently stored nutrient, despite the low carbohydrate mantra that dieters can eat as much fat as they want and continue to lose weight. It sounds too good to be true, and it is. That aside, the evolutionary implications of the "dietary fat isn't stored" claim are spectacular.

If humans were unable to store energy from excess dietary fat, our species would have starved to death at any point in time that carbohydrate became scarce. In cold climates and in winter in general, we would not have been able to survive. Apparently for some low carbohydrate advocates, the human species is either extinct or otherwise has always been able to find carbohydrates in its environment.

All these false claims aside, many dieters have astounding success on low carbohydrate regimens, sometimes losing more than 50 and even more than 100 pounds. These results somewhat skew the value of low carbohydrate diets because people that have 100 or more pounds to lose generally make poor nutritional choices, and an elimination of the carbohydrates in their diets usually means no more pizza, cookies, cakes, and other fast foods. This results in a much better nutritional profile, and a significant reduction in calories.

The impressive 100 pounds lost is the result of eating less and sustaining negative calorie balance for a long enough period of time. The closer you get to your ideal weight, however, the more difficult it becomes to continue getting leaner. The calories have to decrease further, and the hormonal environment of the body has to get even better to keep appetite at bay while maintaining a healthy level of energy expenditure.

Even though the research demonstrates that insulin control by itself is not enough to prevent weight gain or create weight loss, insulin's role in fat gain continues to be a contentious issue. Most diet writers that blame obesity on insulin don't even try to explain how high levels of insulin cause obesity. Many authors simply say insulin is the culprit, relying on the fact that insulin plays a role in fat storage, the end. It is clear that high insulin levels usually accompany weight gain, as do a number of other health problems. However, high insulin levels are not the main cause of weight gain, but are just another symptom of "overeating disease."

That being said, carbohydrate and insulin levels are important when they have an impact on your overall level of energy balance, and this is the situation where overeating elevates insulin levels, and the now higher insulin levels sometimes contribute to further overeating. If you tend to overeat carbohydrates when they are in your diet or if high levels of insulin contribute to your overeating, then macronutrient and hormonal balance can play an important role in your diet.

Decreasing your insulin levels has beneficial health effects and can help weight loss by increasing satiety, but not in the absence of negative energy balance. Manipulating your insulin levels or levels of carbohydrate, while keeping your overall energy intake and energy expenditure constant, will not affect weight loss in any way.[29] Energy balance is first and foremost when it comes to weight loss, and all other hormonal issues should be viewed in the context of their effects on energy balance.

We will explore insulin's role in satiety and overeating in more detail in Chapter 4, Caffeine and Insulin, where we'll discuss how caffeine causes problems for our insulin systems that encourage overeating. Macronutrient and hormonal balance do matter when they affect energy balance, but a wholesale avoidance of carbohydrates is not necessary for most people to achieve their weight loss goals, and insulin control is by far not the only factor that a diet must consider in order to be successful.

Low Fat Diets

At the opposite end of the spectrum from low carbohydrate diets are low fat diets. Low fat dieters correctly point out that fat is the most calorie-dense of the three macronutrients, containing more than twice as many calories per gram than carbohydrates and protein. Low fat dieters also correctly point out that of the three macronutrients, fat is the most efficiently stored as body fat.

Low fat advocates, of course, make some unsupported claims, such as the parallel claim that carbohydrates are never stored as fat, and so forth. Low fat diet writers sometimes claim that only dietary fat can be stored as fat and that carbohydrates will only be used as energy, the opposite of what some low carbohydrate writers claim. Then there are even more radical claims, for example that all animal food is stored as fat or that no foods of vegetable origin are stored as fat, and so on.

Claims such as these are good attention-grabbers, and in cases where they are remotely believable, they are good propaganda. Today we know that all diets work for weight loss when they produce negative energy balance for a long enough period of time. With this knowledge, we can focus on achieving negative energy balance or avoiding positive energy balance in order to achieve and maintain our body composition goals.

The proper focus of a diet is not so much the ratio of macro-nutrients, but the ability to sustain a specific level of energy balance, and macronutrient balance should be evaluated in its ability to maintain the desired level of energy balance. Low fat diets are as effective for fat loss as low carbohydrate diets, so long as they put the individual dieter into negative calorie balance that that individual can maintain for a long enough period of time. If the dieter in question overindulges in low fat and nonfat diet foods to such an extent as to put himself into positive calorie balance, however, he will gain weight regardless of his avoidance of fat.

Very low fat diets are usually difficult to follow because avoiding fat is both difficult and unpleasant for most people. Extremely low fat diets can also cause health problems for the dieter because fat is an essential nutrient and is necessary for health in amounts that vary among individuals. Complete and fanatical avoidance of any one nutrient is not a healthy way to approach dieting in general.

Even in this book, where you will learn that I advocate some reduction and modification of caffeine consumption, I do not advocate complete avoidance, and I do not think complete avoidance of caffeine is practical or enjoyable. Instead, the best way to reduce one's calorie intake is to continue (or begin) to eat a varied diet that does not eliminate any particular nutrient, and to eat small portions of this healthy diet. Eating healthful foods in small amounts is the best solution for lasting weight loss, as long as this creates an energy deficit that can be maintained by the dieter for the time necessary to achieve leanness.

Both low fat diets and low carbohydrate diets work for weight loss when they sufficiently decrease an individual's calorie intake while increasing or maintaining energy expenditure. Due to individual differences that we'll discuss, some people have more success on a low carbohydrate diet, and others have more success on a low fat diet.

In addition to the frameworks of the low carbohydrate and low fat diets, there are a multitude of other diets currently on the market. These run the gamut and include no bread, no grain, Paleolithic, no sugar, no flour, no white food, no yeast, no meat, all meat, no fruit, all fruit, no starch, all starch, all raw, no raw, colorful food only, fasting, and so on, ad infinitum. All of these work to create weight loss when they put you in negative energy balance. So go buy all of them!

Another problem that is common to low carbohydrate, low fat diets, and some other restrictive diets is that these diets often reduce or eliminate foods that are significant sources of healthy nutrients in our diets. Healthy foods are replaced by commercially available "diet" foods that are either low in carbohydrates, low in fat, or low in whatever the dieter is supposed to avoid, depending on the diet in question.

These diet foods are usually highly processed and full of chemicals, so their propriety as a part of any diet is questionable. These restrictive diets are popular, however, and the popularity of macronutrient discrimination for weight loss is partly due to its simplistic approach, and to the ease of building a dietary plan around the elimination of a macronutrient. Completely eliminating a macronutrient such as fat, carbohydrate, or protein helps put the dieter closer to negative calorie balance, tells the dieter what he can and can't eat, and simultaneously obviates the need to count calories.

By eliminating the need to count calories, diets that discriminate against particular foods or macronutrients have helped spread the belief that calories don't matter, a belief that I hope we have adequately put to rest in our discussion of self-reported food intake and the "slow metabolism syndrome."

Dieting Problems

While low calorie diets are the mainstay of obesity treatments, low calorie diets show very modest results in terms of lasting weight loss.[30] In using the term "low caloric diet," I am referring to any diet that works in creating weight loss for some period of time, because by definition, a diet that works must be lower in calories than the regular diet of said dieter. The main reason that many low calorie diets fail is the difficulty most people have in staying on these diets while being hungry.[31] Low calorie diets work for those people who can keep themselves from overeating, and simply do not for those who have difficulty achieving a semblance of satiety.

A comparison of the effects of different popular weight loss diets revealed similar benefits for dieters in terms of weight loss when the dieters stuck to their diets for one year.[32] However, 35-50% of the dieters in this study quit before completing the program, revealing the difficulties of adhering even to the most popular diet plans. Even when dieters are able to stick to a diet for the long run, most of the weight that dieters lose on a diet is regained within 1-3 years, regardless of the type of diet they were originally on.[33] Staying on a diet is made difficult by boredom with the diet and an inability to feel full. Therefore, if we could isolate some ways in which to increase our feelings of fullness and thereby reduce our overeating, it would be much easier to lose weight.

Another problem in dieting is the tedium of counting calories. I won't ask you to count the calories you eat, and I won't ask you to measure your energy expenditure. You can engage in the tedious activity of tallying up your daily food intake, but there is no need to do this. As much as we all like to play with the internet calorie calculators, they can not accurately gauge metabolism with the scant parameters that they ask for, and they can give us false impressions.

Furthermore, your energy expenditure, both at rest and in physical activity, is constantly changing and adjusting itself based on your daily activity levels and nutrition. Instead of counting calories, we should focus changing our diets such that we spontaneously reduce our food intake due to greater levels of satiety. Once a satiety strategy is being employed, the best and most practical way for you to get a sense of your current energy balance is to see if you are losing or gaining weight.

If you are losing weight, you are in negative energy balance. If you are gaining weight, you are in positive energy balance. And if you are neither gaining nor losing weight, then you are in energy balance, with your energy intake and energy expenditure roughly equal. If you have trouble controlling your food intake and are having difficulty reaching a state of undereating, I will try to make this effortless for you.

You will soon learn how not only to speed up your metabolism to increase your chances of undereating and losing weight, but you will also learn how to effortlessly control your appetite simply by manipulating your caffeine intake. Does all of this sound too good to be true? Just you wait and see.

Eat less and exercise more (negative calorie balance) is the central message of most diets that work for weight loss; they just have different methodologies for achieving negative calorie balance. This is the central message of this book as well, but I want to focus on the difficulty in achieving negative calorie balance when consuming caffeine the way we typically consume it. Fortunately, with some more reading and some tweaking of your caffeine intake, negative calorie balance will take care of itself.

Successful Diets

Successful weight loss diets, whether they are low fat diets, low carbohydrate diets, low calorie balanced diets, or any other diets, share some common elements. All diets that produce weight loss do so by putting the dieter in negative calorie balance. They do this by reducing energy intake, by increasing energy expenditure, or both. Successful weight loss diets, once they put the dieter in negative energy balance, are also relatively easy to stay on for the length of time necessary for weight loss to occur. Diets that you can live on for the long-term tend to produce feelings of satiety, so that you are not hungry while dieting.

Negative energy balance and satiety are the most important elements of a weight loss diet. Normal energy balance (neither negative nor positive) and satiety are the most important elements of a diet that maintains your current weight by keeping you from overeating and entering positive energy balance. If we whittle it down even further, we can see that satiety, by itself, is the most important factor of any diet whose goal is to lose weight or keep from gaining it, because feeling full keeps us from overeating.

While other elements such as individual motivation and a lack of boredom are also important to long-term weight loss success, avoiding hunger is more important. Satiety is an interesting phenomenon, because, as we have seen in our above discussion of high protein diets, when dieters achieve satiety, they spontaneously reduce their food intake and lose weight. Satiety is influenced by a number of factors, including an individual's genetics, hormonal profile, and the particulars of the weight loss diet. People experience different degrees of satiety on different diets. Some dieters feel full on low carbohydrate diets, and not on low fat diets, and vice versa. Increased feelings of fullness can make a significant difference in a dieter's ability to sustain a low level of energy balance for the long-term, and these increase feelings of fullness produce better weight loss results.[34]

How do we achieve high levels of satiety? Although it is to some degree an individual phenomenon, satiety is correlated with a high protein intake and with a high fiber intake.[35] As we'll discuss throughout the rest of the book, regular caffeine consumption makes satiety very difficult to achieve. As a result, reducing and modifying your caffeine consumption can produce high levels of satiety and reduce your hunger. In this way, your less-hungry body will spontaneously down-regulate its food intake, just as is the case with high protein and high fiber diets. Your cravings will diminish, you will eat less, and you will lose weight. This principle of satiety, that it causes you to automatically reduce your food intake, is one of the guiding principles of this book.

Besides the satiety principle, successful diets also take advantage of your body's methods of energy expenditure or fat-burning. Both low carbohydrate and low fat diets do this when they shift their dieters' food intake toward high protein and complex carbohydrate foods, respectively. In doing so, they take advantage of the thermic effect and make your body expend more energy in digestion.

In addition, high protein diets help to maintain energy expenditure by maintaining muscle mass. High protein diets can increase energy expenditure due to protein's high thermic effect,[36] and due the maintenance of muscle mass.[37] This is in part due to the fact that the protein needs of the body are higher during negative energy balance as a result of increased muscle breakdown, and an increased protein intake helps to conserve the body's muscle mass while dieters are losing weight.

Higher protein diets are able to conserve more fat-burning muscle tissue and maintain the body's energy expenditure. That being said, some studies do find an energy expenditure advantage of high protein diets and others do not. While some studies find an energy expenditure advantage of high protein diets, when the results of studies that compare different dietary compositions on energy expenditure are averaged, there is no difference between energy expenditure on high carbohydrate and high protein diets.[38] This suggests that both high carbohydrate and high protein diets can sometimes take advantage of the thermic effect or increased muscle maintenance, or both.

We should keep in mind that when studies do find an energy expenditure increase due to a high protein intake, it is found in diets where protein intake is 30-35% of energy intake and the corresponding energy expenditure increase is 70 calories per day for the average adult.[39] This is not a very large increase for the average adult whose daily energy expenditure and required calorie intake are 2500 calories per day, but if we can cut 70 calories here and 70 calories there, the overall impact can be dramatic.

What we should take away from these findings, beyond that of foods' varying thermic effects, is that lean muscle mass is significantly correlated with an individual's metabolic rate at rest.[40] For this reason, a significant portion of this book is concerned with maintaining and increasing your muscle mass, to take advantage of muscle's fat-burning properties, however modest they may be.

Finally, most long-term successful diets prescribe exercise as part of the weight loss lifestyle. Exercise has a very strong protective effect against weight gain because exercise makes it less likely that positive energy balance will occur.[41] Exercise increases dieters' chances of long-term success, so I will talk about incorporating exercise into your routine. If you don't have the time to exercise, however, the caffeine reduction and optimization principles should be enough to get you well on your way to lasting weight loss.

Enter Caffeine

To prevent and treat obesity and create weight loss, energy intake must be reduced, and energy expenditure must be increased. Caffeine is at odds with weight loss because it decreases our feelings of satiety, contributes to overeating, and also decreases our energy expenditure while at rest. By increasing our food intake, caffeine makes lasting leanness and the reversal of weight gain difficult, if not impossible.

The caffeine modification strategies in this book are aimed at decreasing energy intake, increasing energy expenditure, and doing both of these while maintaining high levels of satiety. Satiety is the largest factor in making weight loss sustainable, and so it, and more specifically caffeine's destruction of feelings of satiety, is the largest focus of this book. Modifying your caffeine intake can lead to both a direct spontaneous reduction in your food intake, and also an increase in your resting and active energy expenditures, resulting in significant weight loss and the prevention of weight gain.

Individual Differences

As we will discuss more closely in the next chapter, genetic variations among individuals explain why different people respond to caffeine in different ways.[42] Genetic differences also explain a host of other variations among individuals that are relevant to body composition, including but not limited to, appetite and food cravings, energy expenditure, success on different diets, and so forth.

Researchers often refer to this concept as biochemical individuality, and in the context of caffeine, it explains why one person can have a cup of coffee and feel its effects for hours, while another person won't feel anything at all from one cup, and may need five to feel the same effects. It also partly explains why caffeine is more fattening in some than in others, and takes varying lengths of time to produce its ill effects in different people. I will return to this issue of individual differences throughout the rest of the book, as it comes up again and again in ways that are relevant for our purposes.

While individual differences help to explain why caffeine affects body composition for different individuals differently, let's take a quick look around us. Most Americans consume caffeine on a daily basis, and most Americans have weight problems. These two statements prove nothing of course, because it is just as easy to say that everyone who is overweight breathes air. What I would like to suggest by these statements is that we are not overweight due to a lack of caffeine consumption or even an inadequate level of caffeine consumption. We are not sufferers of caffeine deficiency.

As to the ultra-lean heavy coffee drinker, he is an anomaly, and it may only be a matter of time before caffeine overrides his genetic predisposition toward skinniness. Questioning the role of caffeine in obesity and the weight gain epidemic is long overdue, and my findings may convince you that there is a strong connection between this omni-present drug and our expanding waistlines.

Summary

Your energy balance determines whether you lose or gain weight. The two variables that make up energy balance are energy intake and energy expenditure. Weight gain and obesity are phenomena explained completely by overeating relative to one's energy expenditure and the positive energy balance that is the result. Hormonal balance is important, but only to the extent that it affects energy balance. Macro-nutrient ratios are also important, but only to the extent that they affect energy balance.

In combating overeating and weight gain, the most im-portant weapons are satiety, decreased food intake, and increased physical activity. Caffeine is not an appropriate part of a weight loss diet, because it increases overeating and decreases the body's rate of fat burning while at rest. We'll see how in chapters 3-6. In the next chapter, we'll in-troduce the drug caffeine and the foods and beverages that carry it.

CHAPTER 2
MEET CAFFEINE

It is probably significant that the most widespread words in the world-borrowed into virtually every language-are the names of the four great caffeine plants: coffee, cacao, cola, and tea.

-E.N. Anderson, *The Food of China*, 1988[43]

While I do not want to spend too much time on this section so that we may proceed to the meat of the discussion about caffeine and weight loss, caffeine is interesting enough in and of itself to merit an introduction. If you are more interested in caffeine's fattening properties at the moment, go ahead and skim or skip this chapter and come back when you feel like it. Caffeine's implications for health and body weight are more important for us right now than its history, regardless of how fascinating that history is.

Caffeine

Caffeine is one of a class of compounds called methylxanthines. It was first isolated from coffee by a scientist named Friedlieb Ferdinand Runge in 1819.[44] Runge set out to isolate the chemical responsible for coffee's stimulant effects after a strange encounter with Johann von Goethe, the famous European poet. Goethe set Runge on his path to a shining career in chemistry when he gave Runge a gift of rare coffee beans and suggested that Runge analyze them. The history and development of caffeine as humanity's favorite stimulant is full of strange coincidences like this one, and for the reader who is interested in learning more, I recommend *The World of Caffeine*, written by Bennett Alan Weinberg and Bonnie K. Bealer.

Besides caffeine, the other prominent methylxanthines are theobromine and theophylline.[45] Theobromine and theophylline are present to varying degrees in caffeine-containing beverages and foods. Caffeine is primarily responsible for the effects we feel when we consume coffee, tea, and energy drinks, while theobromine is primarily responsible for the stimulant effects we feel from chocolate.

Caffeine, which can be found in over 60 species of plants, is considered to be the world's most popular drug.[46] People throughout the world have long consumed caffeine from various plant sources including the tea leaf, the coffee bean, cocoa beans, kola nuts, guarana, and maté. All of these caffeine-containing plants were at some point in history used as currency in their respective regions of origin, emphasizing the value that humans placed on these plants from the earliest times of the discovery of their stimulating properties.[47]

Some researchers go so far as to speculate that cavemen discovered many of the caffeine-containing plants as early as 700,000 B.C.E. and chewed on these plants for their stimulant effects.[48] Today, we consume caffeine primarily from coffee, tea, and soft drinks, and do not use caffeine-containing products as currency quite as frequently.[49] It is also interesting to note that all three of these caffeinated beverages were used as medicines when they were first introduced into the human diet.[50] I will briefly introduce these prominent caffeine sources (and chocolate) and then

I will move on to a discussion of caffeine's effects on our minds and bodies.

Tea

Tea is the most appropriate starting point for a discussion of caffeine for at least two reasons. First, tea is second only to water in worldwide consumption. This alone is such an impressive statistic that justifies closely examining the effects of this beverage on human health. Second, it seems that tea is one of the earliest caffeine sources that humankind was able to access.

While accounts of the beginnings of tea consumption differ, there are records that purport to confirm that Chinese consumption of tea in beverage form began as early as the fourth century C.E.[51] The Chinese, perhaps observing the alerting and other psychological effects of the drug, were convinced that tea improved health and prolonged life. It was only many years later, in the seventeenth century, that tea spread to Europe and the British colonies, making its way to what is now the United States.

According to the legend of tea's discovery, Shen Nung, the mythological first emperor of China, was sitting under the shade of a tea bush when he decided to build a fire on which to boil some water. As he was taking some branches from the bush to feed the flames of the fire, the wind blew some of the branch's leaves into the boiling water, giving Shen Nung the first taste of tea and its stimulant effects.

To add to this legend, I will speculate that over time Shen Nung noticed that he could receive a greater stimulant effect from tea if he boiled the leaves longer. The general rule he would have discovered is that the longer tea is brewed, the more caffeine is extracted from the leaves.[52]

Flavors of tea in China vary widely, ranging from mild white teas to sharp green teas to strong-flavored black varieties.[53] Green tea is made from non-oxidized young tea leaves, whereas black tea is made from oxidized leaves. The oxidation process changes the flavor and color of the leaves, and produces leaves with higher caffeine content. Oolong tea is partially oxidized, so it is in the middle of the continuum between green and black tea.

In the United States, we have access to only a small fraction of the varieties of tea, and most of the black tea that we import is used to make iced tea.[54] Tea drinkers and promoters have long attributed health benefits to teas due to their stimulant effects. Today, we attribute the stimulant effect of teas to their caffeine content. The antioxidant activity of tea polyphenols (natural chemical compounds), and not caffeine, is responsible for teas' protective effects against cancer and cardiovascular disease.

Chocolate

Chocolate was the first caffeine-containing food to reach Europe, before tea and coffee. Chocolate has a much lower caffeine content than tea and coffee, but it is the major natural source of theobromine in the human diet. Theobromine is also a stimulant, but a weaker one than caffeine. Theobromine may have a synergistic effect with caffeine, accounting for the distinct stimulant effects of chocolate that produce chocolate cravings.[55]

The cacao tree (the source of chocolate) was cultivated by the Aztec Indians of Mexico and the Maya Indians of Central America since at least the fifth century. The Aztec and Maya prized the plant for its beans and used these beans to make a chocolate drink.[56] After encountering chocolate and its stimulant properties, Cortès brought chocolate to Spain in the sixteenth century. Chocolate then spread throughout Europe where it gradually gained popularity both as a luxury drink and as a medicinal stimulant. The early European chocoholics consumed their chocolate strong, thick and cold, as the Mayans and Aztecs had before them.[57] No doubt most of us today would find the original drink too bitter, and even strange, for our palettes.

Several studies have identified chocolate as the single most craved food, and have suggested that chocolate cravings have a physiological basis. This means that our bodies may develop a liking not only to caffeine, but to theobromine. Today, the chocolate most of us use to satisfy our cravings is milk chocolate, which arrived on the scene in 1876, when it was invented in Switzerland by M.D. Peter. Most of the chocolate we consume is in the form of candy or dessert, rather than in the form of a beverage. The average bar of chocolate contains about six times as much theobromine as caffeine.[58]

There is not much data on the contribution of cocoa and chocolate foods to methylxanthine intake generally and caffeine intake specifically. It is conceivable, however, that for the most hardened chocoholics, who consume the darkest of chocolate in large quantities, these chocoholics receive levels of caffeine comparable to those received by tea and coffee drinkers, in addition to even larger amounts of theobromine.

Coffee

Coffee was late to the caffeine party, with the earliest reliable account of coffee drinking occurring in Yemen in the middle of the fifteenth century.[59] Stepping back from reliable accounts, the legend of the discovery of coffee is that of the Ethiopian goatherd, Kaldi, who supposedly lived in the sixth century. The legend is that Kaldi noticed that his goats had become energized and feisty after chewing on the red berries of a certain bush, so he tried the berries himself, and discovered the coffee bean and its energizing effects. From its mysterious origins, coffee spread via the coffee-house throughout the Middle East and Europe, becoming widespread by the seventeeth century. A sixteenth century coffee lover described coffee as "the common man's gold... bring[ing] to every man the feeling of luxury and nobility.[60] This feeling is pervasive to this day, because coffee is accessible and affordable for everyone.

Coffee was then, as it is now, taken for its stimulant effects. Today, coffee is the primary source of caffeine for most Americans, as well as the most common source of caffeine throughout the world.[61] Even though people drink more tea than coffee in terms of volume, coffee is a more concentrated source of caffeine, being higher in caffeine than tea by about 65%.[62] The American preference for coffee over tea began as a rebellion against all things British after the Boston Tea Party in 1773. In 1774, the Continental Congress even passed a resolution against tea consumption.[63] In effect, it became an American's patriotic duty to drink coffee.

Soft Drinks

Coca-Cola was the first caffeinated soft drink, making its humble debut in the late 19th century as a health tonic sold in pharmacies, and later moving into the broader market. The soft drink's name is derived from the kola nut, which provides one of the flavors of Coca-Cola and a small amount of its caffeine content. Most of the caffeine content in soda comes from caffeine that is the result of tea and coffee de-caffeination. In its early years, Coca-Cola ran into some public relations problems amid concerns that its primary consumers were children, and the soft drink's opponents insisted that children should not be heavy consumers of caffeine.[64]

Coca-Cola resolved this public relations unpleasantness by vowing not to show small children in its advertisements, a vow that it kept until 1986.[65] In an effort to get around this promise and reach its proper target market, the soft drink giant came up with the Coca-Cola-guzzling Santa Claus, who was a huge success in reaching children.[66] Unsurprisingly, coffee has also been marketed to children as young as nine through cartoon characters.[67] Since Coca-Cola invented the soft drink, the market for sweet, carbonated, caffeinated beverages has grown to epic proportions. We will pick up the discussion of soft drinks again in Chapter 5, Addiction-Driven Overeating.

Guarana, Maté, and Medications

Guarana and maté are less common in the American market than they are in other parts of the world, but they are slowly becoming more visible to the American consumer. Guarana is a plant common to South America that produces beans with twice the caffeine content of coffee beans. Traditionally, native South Americans brewed the guarana plant into a tea that they drank for its stimulant effects. Today, guarana is found in soft drinks, energy drinks, and teas that are popular in South America. In the U.S., guarana is found in some teas, energy drinks, and weight loss supplements. Some manufacturers of diet pills like to hide their pills' caffeine content by listing guarana as an ingredient and not listing caffeine, thereby obscuring the consumer's knowledge of the pills' caffeine content.

Maté is also native to South America, and South Americans brew this plant to make a traditional tea. Maté is slowly making its way into the North American tea market and can now increasingly be found not only in loose tea and tea bag form, but also in bottled form. I have begun to see different flavors of maté available in natural retailers such as Whole Foods Market. It is also beginning to make its way into soda. The caffeine content of maté is similar to that of tea, and it remains to be seen how far into the North American caffeinated beverage market this plant will penetrate.

Medications, both prescription and non-prescription, are yet another source of caffeine in the diet. The primary uses of these caffeine-containing medications are pain relief, alertness, weight loss, and cough and cold relief.[68] Compared to coffee, tea, soft drink, and chocolate consumption, caffeine intake from medications is not significant for most of the population. However, if you take large amounts of caffeine pills for energy or aspirin-caffeine combination pills for headaches, your caffeine intake from these pills can be quite high.

This ends our discussion of the sources of caffeine in the human diet. It has by no means been an exhaustive list of all the caffeine sources in the human diet, but it adequately describes the prevalent caffeine sources in the United States.

Stimulant as Yardstick

In Norway, distances were once measured in "coffee boils," the number of times a traveler needed to prepare coffee along the way.[69] This is similar to the use of coca leaves in South America. The coca leaf is the natural source of cocaine, and South Americans chew the leaf for its stimulant effects. In areas where the leaf is chewed, travelers sometimes measure distances by "cocada," the distance that can be traveled on one chew.[70] This is arguably neither here nor there, but I think it emphasizes the centrality of stimulants in society. In the United States, we also use caffeine to measure time when we talk about how long we can last on one cup of coffee until we need another to remain productive at our daily tasks. Some of us who use caffeine to get through school and work assignments measure the impressiveness of a project by the amount of caffeine that we consumed to complete it, so caffeine's use as a measuring device is present even in the United States.

Caffeine Statistics

According to recent studies, approximately 90% of people use caffeine consistently, and the exact figure may be even higher.[71] In the U.S., it is estimated that over 80% of adults consume caffeine on a daily basis, with the bulk of our consumption coming from coffee, tea, and soft drinks.[72] Per capita consumption of caffeine averages 200 mg/day, the equivalent of two cups of coffee.[73] Caffeine use is not limited to adults, as studies demonstrate that 98% of children consume caffeine at least once a week. The major source of caffeine for children is tea, followed by soda and chocolate. Chocolate provides less than 20% of a child's caffeine intake.[74] When children are exposed to a combination of tea, soda, and chocolate in their diets, they can easily consume up to 200 mg of caffeine per day, as adults do. Furthermore, one serving of caffeinated soda, which contains about 50 mg of caffeine, may have the same biological and physiological effects in a child as 2 cups of coffee in an adult.[75] If a child consumes 200 mg of caffeine, that child is consuming the adult equivalent of 8 cups of coffee.

That's something to think about, considering that in recent years, coffeehouses have become more successful in attracting young customers, usually in their early teens.[76] If this pattern continues, coffee may gain more ground as a beverage consumed by children and teenagers. Regardless of when an individual's caffeine consumption begins, from that point caffeine consumption increases as an individual gets older until it stabilizes around middle age.[77] As a society we are beginning to take up caffeine earlier in our lives than previously, and generally once we begin our caffeine intake, we don't stop it.

Caffeine in the Body

After an individual consumes caffeine, blood levels of the drug reach their peak within an hour of ingestion, and the body removes most of the caffeine within twelve hours. The rate at which individuals eliminate caffeine varies according to a number of lifestyle, genetic, and nutritional factors. Among healthy adults, there is as much as a five fold variation in the rates at which they eliminate caffeine. Other drugs affect the rate of caffeine metabolism. Smoking increases the rate at which caffeine is eliminated, while alcohol and oral contraceptives reduce the rate at which caffeine is eliminated.[78]

Genetic differences explain why some people have stronger physiological and psychological reactions to caffeine than other people.[79] Genetic differences also explain people's preferences and responses to caffeine. In fact, people's varied responses to the drug may be modified over time by caffeine use itself.[80] A person's response to caffeine may weaken, strengthen, become better, or become worse over time. There is also some anecdotal evidence that different sources of caffeine have different effects for certain individuals. For example, some people feel nothing after having several cups of coffee, but just one cup of tea makes these people bounce off the walls. At this point we do not know the reason for this response but I suppose it may be in part psychological and in part due to the different methylxanthine combinations present in coffee and tea.

Genetic factors also affect the rate at which an individual eliminates caffeine.[81] For example, some people, who are "slow acetylators," have livers that are genetically slow to eliminate caffeine and as a result are more sensitive to the drug's effects. A large portion of the population may be slow to eliminate caffeine. One study that evaluated the rate of caffeine elimination of 595 healthy volunteers found that 61.7% of the group was slow to acetylate caffeine.[82]

If this can be generalized to the larger population, then it is possible that most of the population is slow to eliminate caffeine. The longer that the caffeine is present in our bodies, the longer its effects last, including those that encourage weight gain. Nutritional factors are also important because healthy acetylation is dependent on having adequate levels of thiamine, pantothenic acid, and vitamin C. When these nutrients are low, the elimination of caffeine is slowed, and its effects in the body last longer. In the above-described ways, lifestyle, genetic, and nutritional factors help explain why the same cup of coffee will have different effects for different people.

At the Workplace

Caffeine consumption at work through coffee and tea drinking has a long history. Much of our daily intake of caffeine occurs on the job, where it is commonly used in an effort to improve mental performance. We assume that the ubiquitous office coffee pot is heavily used by workers in order to increase their levels of wakefulness, alertness, and, more generally, productivity. There may, however, be some other benefits of caffeine intake in the office setting. Headaches, for example, are often reported in work settings, and one study showed that workers sometimes consume caffeine primarily to relieve their headaches. This discovery is consistent with the widespread medical use of caffeine to treat headaches.[83]

Another common reason for caffeine consumption in the office setting is boredom.[84] The mood lift many of us associate with caffeine helps to relieve this on-the-job boredom. Caffeinated beverages give us a mood lift in part because caffeine stimulates the release of serotonin in the brain.[85] Serotonin is a neurotransmitter that contributes to feelings of well-being. In addition to serotonin, caffeine also stimulates the release of dopamine, another neurotransmitter that is also associated with pleasure and feelings of well-being. The effects of these two neurotransmitters in the human brain are in part responsible for the mood-improving effects we often experience when we consume caffeinated beverages and foods.

Spiders

Plants developed the ability to produce caffeine because it acts as a pesticide, protecting the plants from insects and harmful single-celled organisms.[86] Ironically, caffeine-producing plants ultimately succumb to the harmful effects of caffeine themselves. As the caffeine-producing plant thrives, the soil around it gradually becomes rich with caffeine from the plant's falling leaves and fruit. Over time, the caffeine in the soil surrounding a caffeine-producing plant reaches a level of caffeine concentration high enough to poison the plant itself. This self-poisoning is one of the main reasons for the degeneration of coffee plantations over time.[87]

An interesting experiment performed by NASA scientists sought to determine the toxicity of various chemicals by exposing spiders to these chemicals and then measuring the extent to which the spiders' web-spinning ability was altered by each chemical. The chemical which produced the most deformation in the spiders' webs was caffeine.[88] The idea of this testing is to extrapolate the results and determine the toxicity of various chemicals not to spiders but to humans. However, it is difficult to extrapolate the data in this way when the chemical (caffeine) in question developed in nature as a pesticide, so its effects in spiders are likely to be completely different than its effects in humans, being that spiders are one of caffeine's intended targets. That being said, Spiderman, if you're reading this, take note, as it may explain why your journalism suffers so greatly after your morning cup of coffee.

Caffeine Content Reference

Before we move on to caffeine's fattening properties, here are three tables that show the caffeine content of various beverages and foods, soft drinks in some depth, and medications in some depth, respectively. This quick reference is intended for both humans and spiders.

Caffeine Content of Various Beverages and Foods[89]		
Beverage	Serving/volume	Caffeine (mg)
Coffee		
Automatic drip	5 oz	115 (80-175)
Percolated	5 oz	80 (40-170)
Instant	5 oz	60 (46-71)
Espresso	1.5-2 oz	100
Cappuccino	6 oz	60-120
Decaffeinated	6 oz	<5
Tea	6 oz	30-80
Iced	12 oz	70
Brewed, imported	7 oz	60
Brewed, U.S.	7 oz	40
Chocolate		
Chocolate milk	8 oz	2-8
Hot chocolate	8 oz	10
Milk chocolate	1 oz	6
Dark chocolate	1 oz	20
Chocolate cake	1 slice	20-30

Caffeine Content of some Cola Beverages[90]	
Beverage Name	Caffeine Content (mg/12 fl oz)
Cherry Coca-Cola®	46
Diet Cherry, Coca-Cola®	46
Cherry Cola Slice®	48
Diet Cherry Cola Slice®	41
Coca-Cola®	46
Diet Coke®, Coca-Cola®	46
Coca-Cola Classic®	46
Dr. Pepper®	41
Diet Dr. Pepper®	41
Mr. Pibb®	40
Pepsi Cola®	38
Diet Pepsi®	36
Pepsi Lite®	36
Diet Rite Cola®	48
7UP Gold®	46
Diet 7UP Gold®	46
Tab®	46
Diet cola, aspartame sweetened	50
Diet soda, sodium saccharin sweetened	39
Jolt	100
Mountain Dew	54

Selected Prescription and Non-Prescription Medications Containing Caffeine [91]		
Medications	Dose	Caffeine (mg)
Analgesics/pain relief		
Excedrin	2 tablets	130
Anacin	2 tablets	64
Midol	2 tablets	64
Midol, Max Strength	1 tablet	60
Cafergot	1 tablet	100
Darvon	2 tablets	60
Fioricet with codeine	1 tablet	40
Fiorinal	1 tablet	40
Norgesic	1 tablet	30
Norgesic Forte	1 tablet	60
Vanquish	1 tablet	33
Decongestants		
Dristan decongestant	2 tablets	32
Stimulants		
NoDoz	1 dose	200
Vivarin	1 dose	200
Weight loss		
Dexatrim	1 dose	200

Summary

A variety of plants produce caffeine as an insecticide. At various points in history, people began to discover that the various caffeine-containing plants had stimulating properties when their leaves, fruits, and other parts were chewed or consumed as tea. Once the pleasant effects of caffeine were known, the popularity of this stimulant spread throughout the world. Today, the most common sources of caffeine are tea, coffee, soft drinks, and chocolate.

Most of us consume caffeine on a daily basis, especially as a wakefulness aid in the morning and productivity aid at work. Once we develop our caffeine habits, most of us keep these habits for life. A number of genetic, nutritional, and lifestyle factors explain the diverse physiological effects of caffeine among different individuals. In the next chapter we will finally begin our discussion of caffeine's fattening properties.

CHAPTER 3
CAFFEINE AND
CORTISOL

It's the devil's nectar. It's filthy and unhealthy.
-Mark Helprin, *Memoir from Antproof Case*, referring to coffee (1995)

Cortisol commands a lot of attention in the weight loss marketplace and there are a number of products which promise to help the individual dieter lose weight by lowering and controlling her cortisol levels. Whole books are written about cortisol. So what is cortisol? Is it important for weight loss? And if it is, then why?

Cortisol is a steroid hormone produced by the adrenal glands. Fasting, exercise, awakening, certain foods, and physical and psychological stress all cause the body to release cortisol.[92] Our cortisol levels increase when we encounter any event, whether physical or psychological, that causes us to feel stress. Even imagined stress, such as thinking about a possible conflict at work, will raise our cortisol levels.

As a result of its production in response to physical and psychological stress, cortisol has become known as the "stress hormone." Stress can be described as a feeling of being overcome by the events in your life. We all know people who get stressed out over little things and others who are undaunted in the face of even the most overwhelming circumstances. People have varying levels of stress tolerance, and cortisol levels vary accordingly.

Once the body produces cortisol in response to one of life's stressors, its function is to provide us with the energy we need to respond to that stressor. The cortisol response includes the mobilization of energy stores for immediate use, the relocation of the body's fat stores, increased hunger, and muscle breakdown.

Caffeine consumption results in an increased production of cortisol in the body, even in those individuals who are habitual caffeine consumers and whose bodies have presumably adapted to caffeine.[93] So even if you are a regular coffee drinker and you no longer get much stimulation from your coffee, you still do get an increase in your levels of stress hormones.

Researchers have also demonstrated that caffeine consumption results in elevated cortisol levels both when it is consumed by itself in a relaxed environment and when consumed under stress. This is an extremely important consideration for individuals who are trying to lose weight or maintain a lean physique, as cortisol has strong effects on appetite, your resting energy expenditure (metabolism), and the location of fat stores.

Many people blame their weight gain on high levels of stress, and they are right. Chronic stress results in a chronically elevated cortisol level, which is one of the most significant contributing factors to increased appetite, overeating, and muscle breakdown that leads to a lower resting energy expenditure.

I would even go so far as to say that caffeine is one of the primary stressors in modern society, increasing our cortisol levels and keeping them elevated when we should not otherwise be stressed. Studies report that dietary doses of caffeine are capable of producing the same cortisol response as mental and physiological stress, and can exacerbate the cortisol response when an individual is already confronting non-dietary stress.

Lions, Tigers, Bears, and Caffeine

The evolutionary purpose of the stress response is to prepare us to fight or flee from a predator. This is why we often refer to it as the fight-or-flight response. In other words, the body gathers its energy to enable us to try to run away from a bear or any other large and hungry animal. Before the advent of modern society, if we were successful in outrunning the bear, or more likely in outrunning one of our slower compatriots, our stress levels would fall back to normal when we caught our breath and calmed down.

In modern times, however, due to the way we structure our lives and due to certain dietary habits such as regular caffeine use, our bodies are constantly in this frantic fight-or-flight state. We are always running from the bear. While our bodies have evolved to deal with short-lived intermittent stressors (occasional hungry predators), they have not had nearly as much time to adjust to the continuous stress and continuously elevated cortisol levels that we experience today.

Two hundred milligrams of caffeine, the amount found in two cups of coffee, can increase your blood cortisol levels by thirty percent within one hour![94] This is a large contribution to elevated cortisol levels. A wide range of research has shown that chronically elevated cortisol levels (and therefore stress levels) are associated with weight gain, leading many researchers to suspect a causal connection between the two.

The negative health effects associated with high cortisol levels include obesity, binge eating, high blood pressure, diabetes, fatigue, depression, moodiness, and a decreased sex drive.[95] Women respond more strongly to stress than men, meaning that women experience a greater increase in cortisol levels than men when facing similar stressors.[96] Women also eliminate caffeine more slowly than men, and more slowly still if they use oral contraceptives.

As a result, women who consume caffeine regularly may find themselves more susceptible to chronically elevated cortisol levels, and the associated weight gain, than men. While consistently high levels of cortisol are undesirable, a certain amount of this hormone is necessary for health, so this chapter describes the dangers of chronically elevated cortisol levels, and does not advocate a complete elimination of cortisol in the body.

Many healthcare professionals are now acknowledging the role stress plays in the accumulation of body fat. Some of the leading researchers of stress, cortisol and obesity recommend a reduction of caffeine and other stimulants as one of the most significant anti-stress decisions an individual can make.[97] This is logical because caffeine is one of the main factors in modern life, and possibly *the* main factor, that contributes to chronic stress.

By limiting caffeine, not only can you improve your body composition, but your stress levels may decrease to such a degree as to make you feel like a whole new person. When I stay away from caffeine consistently, I feel a strong sense of calm at all times. When I stray from the caffeine-free path, however, I begin to feel frazzled, anxious, and progressively more stressed. For many people, stress-induced overeating is a huge factor in their struggles to lose weight, and as we will discuss in a moment, stress-induced overeating is biologically driven.

A Bigger Appetite

There are studies that suggest the mechanism by which cortisol encourages overeating is by making us resistant to leptin.[98] Leptin is a hormone that monitors and maintains the body's energy balance, and can be described as the hunger hormone. Leptin regulates appetite by either promoting appetite or suppressing appetite, depending on what it determines is going on in the body.

If leptin levels are low in the body, or if we become resistant to leptin, we lose control of our appetites and become prone to overeating. In healthy individuals, if leptin is present, then appetite is suppressed. By making our bodies resistant to the effects of leptin, however, chronically elevated cortisol levels keep our appetites going strong when we are actually full and should not be hungry. Low leptin levels and reduced sensitivity to leptin make weight gain, and weight regain after weight loss, more likely.[99]

Leptin is supposed to tell us that we have adequate fat stores and should reduce our food consumption. It is also supposed to tell us that we are full after we eat, so we don't keep eating. That's how our bodies regulate themselves and why people who are healthy never need to count calories.

For a number of dietary and lifestyle reasons, it seems that the majority of the U.S. population has issues with leptin resistance, having become insensitive to the effects of this hunger-curbing hormone. Cortisol is not the only culprit, and we will revisit leptin in Chapter 5, Addiction-Driven

Overeating, where we will see that dietary sugar has a similar negative effect on leptin sensitivity, as cortisol does.

Regardless of the exact biological mechanisms involved, chronically elevated cortisol levels promote overeating and bring on cravings for calorie-dense foods.[100] Several studies have demonstrated that high cortisol levels are associated with increased appetite, cravings for fat and sugar, and weight gain. There is now evidence that stress causes us to undereat in the beginning of the stress response, and then to overeat in the later stages of the stress response, which can last from hours to days.

So when we drink coffee, we may feel our appetite suppressed for a little while (the period of time in which we should be making our getaway from a hungry predator), but then our appetite comes back with a vengeance and can stay elevated for days. This is not a desirable tradeoff if your goal is weight loss or the maintenance of a lean physique.

From an evolutionary perspective, the increased appetite makes perfect sense because after the presumed stress of running away from a predator, the body seeks to replace the energy that it has expended in completing the getaway. When you overeat because you feel stressed, it's not "all in your head." None of it is. The increased appetite you feel and your desire to overeat is not a function of having insufficient willpower. It is a biologically driven response that the human body has learned and that has historically helped us to survive.

Some studies have shown that overweight and obese individuals overproduce cortisol in response to food when compared to lean individuals, and also exhibit hardier cortisol levels when given cortisol-suppressing drugs.[101] A recent study found that obese children had higher cortisol levels than normal, suggesting a link between elevated cortisol levels and obesity.[102] Researchers who conducted another study on binge eating found that women who are binge eaters have higher levels of cortisol than is normal, and noted that stress is the most commonly reported trigger for binge eating.[103]

If we can remove or reduce the contribution that caffeine makes to our stress levels, we can expect a corresponding decrease in our binge eating behaviors and overeating generally. This reduced food intake can go a very long way in creating weight loss and preventing further weight gain. The above studies associate cortisol with overeating, and the studies in the preceding paragraphs suggest a strong causal link between cortisol and increased appetite and overeating. With this large amount of research support, cortisol's role in overeating can not be ignored.

Less Muscle

The effects of a chronically elevated cortisol level, in addition to increased appetite and a tendency to overeat, include muscle breakdown, which reduces our rates of energy expenditure while at rest.[104] Cortisol also slows down our metabolic rates by decreasing levels of thyroid stimulating hormone (TSH), and we will revisit this issue in Chapter 6, Diet Pills, Green Tea, and the Thyroid, in which we'll uncover the inefficacy of caffeine-containing weight loss supplements and question the health benefits of consuming large amounts of green and black tea.

Chronically elevated cortisol levels mobilize the body's energy reserves to deal with a stressor (by running away), and depress levels of testosterone, growth hormone, and DHEA, resulting in a breakdown of muscle and bone tissue and the promotion of fat gain.[105] Testosterone, growth hormone, and DHEA are all important for building and maintaining your body's muscle mass. DHEA is a sex hormone produced in the adrenal glands which is then converted to testosterone, estrogen, progesterone, or cortisol, depending on the body's needs at the time.[106]

The more cortisol that our bodies produce, the less DHEA we are left with for other tasks, including the creation of muscle-promoting testosterone. If we can successfully control our production of cortisol, then we will conserve more of our DHEA levels for use in testosterone creation. As we discussed in the first chapter, it is our fat-free mass in the form of muscle that is most directly related to our rate of energy expenditure while at rest.

Cortisol decreases resting energy expenditure by breaking down muscle, and thereby reducing the total amount of fat-burning muscle mass an individual carries.[107] Muscle breakdown is one of the ways that cortisol mobilizes the body's energy, by breaking down our muscle protein and converting it into immediately usable amino acids and glucose to fuel our presumed getaway from a predator.[108] Elevated cortisol levels can increase the rate of muscle breakdown in the body by 5-20%.[109]

Research has shown that even mild increases in cortisol can increase muscle breakdown in healthy individuals within a few hours.[110] For this reason, bodybuilders especially revile and fear cortisol. It is interesting to note here that despite the negative consequences of a high caffeine intake for a bodybuilder's muscle conservation purposes, Vivarin, a nonprescription caffeine pill, is actively marketed to bodybuilders, promising better alertness and concentration in the weight room.[111]

Our cortisol levels increase as we age, and this may in part explain why we become fatter and less muscular as we get older.[112] This also coincides with the caffeine consumption pattern we discussed in the previous chapter, which indicates that people increase their caffeine consumption as they get older until their caffeine consumption stabilizes in middle age. Cortisol breaks down muscle and increases appetite, so it is no surprise that as the levels of this hormone increase in our bodies, we gain weight.

As we age, our resting energy expenditures slow due to the muscle loss we experience as a result of our caffeine consumption, other sources of stress, disuse, poor diet, and the changing hormonal environment that accompanies aging. For every ten years that we age, we burn approximately five percent fewer calories per day due in part to our declining muscle mass, and this decreased ability to burn fat can add up in terms of fat storage.[113] A lack of resistance training aside, at least some of the age-related muscle loss we experience can be explained by chronically elevated cortisol levels from chronic caffeine consumption.

Coffee Belly

Prolonged exposure to elevated levels of cortisol also results in the relocation of fat from deposits throughout the body to deep within and around the abdomen, resulting in higher levels of visceral fat, which is the fat surrounding our internal organs.[114] Elevated cortisol levels tell your body to store fat preferentially in and around your abdomen. We will discuss further hormonal implications of visceral fat in the next chapter, but for now let's focus on the aesthetic implications of visceral fat.

For cortisol to shape one's body, cortisol levels must be elevated for an extended period of time, as is the case with chronic caffeine consumption. Furthermore, for cortisol to shape one's body, ideally the stressor, in this case caffeine, will produce elevated cortisol levels indefinitely. This condition is satisfied because the cortisol response to caffeine does not decline with continued caffeine use, as we discussed above. We do not develop a tolerance to the cortisol-raising effects of caffeine, and it is able to change the shape of our bodies in an unflattering manner.

By increasing levels of general central fat and visceral fat, cortisol damages an individual's appearance. This deep-in-the-body visceral fat accumulation causes the belly to stick out prominently, creating what some refer to as "coffee belly." This unattractive state is most often referred to as "beer belly" or "beer gut," because of its high rate of incidence among beer enthusiasts.

Unsurprisingly, the mechanism that creates a beer belly is the same mechanism that creates a coffee belly, because alcohol also raises the body's cortisol levels. From an evolutionary perspective, relocating fat stores to the center of the body and the abdominals depths may have had significant purposes.

In moving fat stores from their deposits around the body to its center, cortisol helps ensure that in future stressful situations, fat is available for rapid mobilization, as fat is easier to burn from the center of the body where there is the most blood flow. In addition, by signaling your body to store fat around your organs, cortisol ensures that your organs have a protective cushion of fat for the inevitable fall in one of your flights from a predator.

As a result, you will be less likely to suffer an organ-damaging injury, which may threaten your survival. The more cortisol the body is exposed to on a regular basis, the greater is the signal that the body is constantly under stress. The relocation of fat that results is the body's way of recognizing chronic stress and preparing to deal with the ongoing stress in an efficient manner.

Although a high level of overall fat is usually accompanied by high levels of visceral and central fat, this is not always the case. Sometimes central fat levels and overall fat levels can uncouple, giving an overweight individual a relatively narrow waist and giving a lean individual a relatively thick waist.[115]

Furthermore, a relatively lean individual with high levels of central fat may be at particular risk for central fat's associated health problems. There is a significant genetic component to the location of fat stores, so some regular coffee drinkers may not find their midsections expanding as much as others do. If you are already genetically predisposed to central fat storage, however, chronically elevated cortisol levels will make your central fat storing tendency more pronounced.

Spot Addition

Spot reduction is the notion that certain exercises can reduce fat in specific areas on the body. For example, some exercisers believe that crunches take fat off the abdominals, and that leg exercises take fat off the thighs. Whether spot reduction is possible is a hotly debated issue in the fitness community. Most of the fitness writers call it a myth. However, even though I do not want to get pulled into this controversy, I will state that the evidence on the topic is not yet conclusive. But I don't want to talk about spot reduction anyway. What I want to talk about is spot addition!

The belief in spot reduction may be unfounded, but when it comes to the addition of fat to our bodies, it is true that we tend to add it to certain places more than others. And while there is a strong genetic component that determines where your body fat will go, there is also a dietary component.

Cortisol directs more of your fat to be stored centrally, and caffeine intake and your diet in general will influence your cortisol level. Caffeine makes spot addition of fat to your middle a reality.

As I myself experienced, a protruding belly can be especially ruinous on a skinny person with a small frame. Having relatively narrow shoulders will add to the prominence of a large belly, and thereby destroy the body's aesthetics. A term I sometimes hear to describe a small-framed individual with a gut is "skinny fat." The term is appropriate because skinny fat individuals are not large enough to be called fat, but their small bodies are overshadowed by a disproportionate belly.

This is the body type that researchers describe as being most indicative of serious health problems down the road. So not only was my skinny fatness unattractive and crushing to my self-esteem, but it came with a number of serious health implications. Stopping your body from relocating fat to the depths of your belly will improve your appearance markedly, and will help you fit into those old jeans, or in my case, dress pants, that you have hanging in the closet.

Central fat storage is unattractive by contemporary aesthetic standards, which emphasize a trim waist. That is an understatement. In our ab-obsessed society, having a small, lean midsection is paramount in creating an attractive physique. Although notions of symmetry and the most attractive amount of body fat change over time, we need to work with what we have right now, and the current ideal body type is a thin, trim-waisted one. In trying to come closer to this aesthetic ideal then, it is preferable to keep fat stores more evenly distributed throughout the body, rather than have these fat stores moved to within and around the waist, creating the coffee belly and spare tire effects.

I am concerned not only with making you healthier, but also with making you leaner and thereby more attractive. I also believe that attractiveness and health are inextricably linked, so in improving one (through natural means of course), we improve the other - not to mention the effects on your self-esteem and confidence that improving your appearance can have.

If you are like most individuals, the fastest way to move your appearance toward aesthetic symmetry is by narrowing your waist. I would rather keep my fat spread out, and I do not mind having some of my fat stored in my muscles as intramuscular fat, (and perhaps this fat can even serve to give me a meaner appearance). What I do not want is for cortisol to relocate this fat from inside my muscles, where it is not as aesthetically displeasing, to my midsection, the prime spot for fat to provide aesthetic displeasure.

If all of the above is not enough to drive home the point that we need to focus on keeping our visceral fat to a healthy minimum, high levels of visceral fat also put individuals at greater risk of developing type 2 diabetes, cardiovascular disease, high blood pressure, and high cholesterol. We will leave our discussion of visceral fat on this point, but we will return to this discussion in the next chapter, when we examine how this accumulation of visceral fat also harms the insulin sensitivity of the body's tissues and further contributes to weight gain.

The next point in our parade of horribles is fluid retention. There is a possibility that elevated levels of cortisol also contribute to fluid retention by causing the body to hold on to sodium.[116] This is problematic because even though fluid is not fat, it still creates the appearance of fat or a slightly different "puffy" look, which can make you look bigger and carry more weight around with you.

However, the extent of this fluid retention is uncertain due to caffeine's diuretic (water expelling) effect, so if we subtract caffeine's diuretic effect from the cortisol-induced fluid retention, what we are left with probably varies on an individual basis. The jury is still out on caffeine's net effect on fluid retention, although most sources suggest that caffeine is helpful for getting excess fluid out of the body.

Fresh Fruits and Vegetables

Vitamin C is one of the most important vitamins for controlling stress levels and as such it is usually included in stress-reducing supplements. This vitamin decreases stress by helping to normalize cortisol levels.[117] I do not take vitamin or mineral supplements myself, so I am not one to recommend them. However, I love fresh fruits and vegetables, and I have no problem recommending those to everyone (assuming you are not allergic to the ones I recommend). In order to keep up my own levels of vitamin C, I eat citrus fruits, berries, and fresh greens such as romaine and spinach.

There is value in treating stress with diet, and I recommend that you eat a variety of fresh fruits and vegetables to help combat stress and keep your cortisol levels in line. If you regularly include these foods in your diet then you are already doing a lot to keep your stress levels down and to obtain any other metabolic benefits of fresh fruits and vegetables (new benefits are being discovered all the time). If fruits and vegetables are not a regular part of your diet, you might feel a big downward shift in your stress levels and an upward shift in your overall sense of well-being when you begin to include these foods.

In general, the more stress you are experiencing at a given time, the more important nutritional support becomes. So if work is being especially stressful, you may want to add a few extra oranges and salads to your menu. You will also find that by keeping high levels of cortisol at bay, these foods reduce your hunger and help keep you from overeating.

Additive Effects

Caffeine consumption has negative effects in the workplace as an aggravator of pre-existing and new on-the-job stressors.[118] Caffeine has an additive effect when it is consumed at work such that our stress response to work events is higher than it would be if we were not consuming caffeine. This effect is particularly visible in caffeine's impact on our blood pressure. Caffeine increases both resting blood pressure and the blood pressure response to stress. Other studies have shown that workers become more prone to psychological stress after consuming caffeine, so in effect these workers feel that they are under more pressure to perform.

A number of studies also demonstrate that caffeine use increases anxiety and feelings of anxiety, and this anxiety-inducing property presents itself in both habitual users as well as non-users, suggesting that a tolerance to this negative effect does not develop with habitual use. The anxiety-producing and aggravating effects of caffeine have been observed in children as young as 8 years old, and males are more sensitive to this effect than females.[119]

One study determined that caffeine increases the stress response of military recruits in a combat setting. The researchers who performed the study recommended that the use of decaffeinated coffee may help to reduce combat stress and other anxiety reactions in a military setting.[120] Yet another study determined that caffeine ingestion more than doubled the stress response to a demanding task, and habitual caffeine consumers were not immune to this increase in stress.[121] The stress-increasing effects of caffeine do not go away with habitual use, and it is likely that most of us have experienced these effects in stressful settings.

Stress experts contend that we experience a consistently high level of stress because we lead hectic lives and get less than eight hours of sleep per night.[122] To these already stressful circumstances we add a dietary stimulant in the form of caffeine, which builds upon and exacerbates our existing stress levels. Caffeine lowers the body's stress threshold, so that everyday events become more stressful for us than they otherwise would be.

After a period of stress, cortisol remains elevated even after five days of rest following the stressful event, and it may take as long as three weeks after the removal of a stressor such as caffeine for our cortisol levels to return to normal.[123] This means that even after we stop or reduce our caffeine consumption, it will take some time for our bodies to down-regulate cortisol production for us to see the positive health effects of lower stress levels.

A Horse of Course!

Stress and high cortisol levels result in a reduced sex drive in both men and women.[124] The reduction in sex drive is explained by cortisol's testosterone-depressing effects. Testosterone is vital for a healthy sex drive and muscle maintenance in both men and women. Furthermore, sex does burn calories, and I have even seen it recommended as a method for maintaining one's physical fitness (probably on a daytime talk show). Also, having an interest in sex no doubt motivates people to remain attractive by keeping their weight under control. In these two admittedly indirect ways, maintaining a high sex drive can help you attain and keep a lean body. The real reason I bring up sex drive, however, is to lead into the following coffee legend, which reiterates the fact that people have questioned the health effects of caffeine-containing beverages from the moment these beverages took over the world.

The relevant legend describes a coffee-loving king of Persia who consumed so much of the beverage that he lost all interest in his wife. The wife then apparently made a connection between the king's coffee drinking and his nonexistent sex drive. Soon afterwards, while she was lounging about bemoaning her mislaid sex life, the king's wife inquired about a stallion that was being castrated; asking what was being done to the poor horse. When she learned that the intent was to cure the horse of lust, she replied that the horse need not be castrated, as all that was needed was to feed the horse coffee, and he would become like the king.[125]

Apparently the queen in the above legend was not alone in her observations. In London in 1674, some disgruntled women got together and drafted *The Women's Petition Against Coffee*, complaining that coffee has so "*Eunucht* our Husbands, and *Crippled* our more kind *Gallants*... [that] They come from it with nothing *moist* but their snotty Noses, nothing *stiffe* but their Joints, nor *standing* but their Ears."[126] Poor women! Both of these accounts, if somewhat exaggerated, remind us that people have questioned the effects of caffeine, in this case its effects on virility, for centuries.

Summary

Caffeine raises your body's cortisol levels and keeps them elevated. Caffeine also increases your body's stress response to other physiological and psychological stressors such as job stress. Chronically elevated cortisol levels contribute to overeating, to muscle breakdown, and to the relocation of fat stores to the center of your body. Cortisol-induced over-eating and muscle breakdown help to put your body in, or closer to, positive energy balance, making you gain weight or have more difficulty losing it. Cortisol-induced fat store relocation helps create the "coffee belly" look which ruins the body's aesthetic symmetry and efforts to create and maintain a narrow waist.

Besides the caffeine reduction strategies that will be de-scribed later in the book, the best way to keep your cortisol levels in check and keep your levels of stress under control is by adopting and maintaining a diet that is high in fresh fruits and vegetables. In the next chapter, we will discuss another way that caffeine causes us to overeat; by making us crave starchy and sugary foods.

CHAPTER 4
CAFFEINE AND
INSULIN

Man does not live by coffee alone. Have a Danish.

-Anonymous

Cortisol is not the only hormone that caffeine use affects. Caffeine also raises insulin levels and contributes both to insulin resistance and reactive hypoglycemia, each of which presents problems when a dieter is trying to keep from overeating.[127] While high insulin levels do not cause fat gain on their own, high insulin levels can significantly increase our tendency to overeat. Before delving into these problems, let's first become better acquainted with glucose and insulin.

Glucose is a simple sugar that is the body's primary source of energy. The body receives glucose from carbohydrate-rich foods. Carbohydrates can be found in a variety of starchy and sugary foods such as bread, pasta, potatoes, rice, corn, fruit, sugar, honey, and sweets. All carbohydrates are broken down into simple sugars through digestion, unless they are already simple sugars when they enter the body. After the digestion of starches and sugars, glucose enters the bloodstream. As a result, blood glucose levels rise and this rise signals cells in the pancreas to produce insulin.

Insulin's function is to escort glucose from the blood into the cells that require it for energy and energy storage. In a healthy body, insulin efficiently brings glucose to cells, reducing the level of glucose in the blood as it does so, and blood glucose is maintained within a narrow range. Insulin transports glucose to cells for immediate energy use, for storage as glycogen, and for storage as fat. Insulin also inhibits a hormone called glucagon, which has the opposite function of insulin in that it raises glucose levels in the blood by releasing stored energy from the liver, muscle, and fat cells.

Because one of insulin's functions is fat storage, many diet writers like to vilify insulin by calling it a "storage hormone," and suggesting that insulin is what makes us fat. This is a gross oversimplification, given that insulin also delivers glucose for immediate energy use and for storage as glycogen, which is not fat. It is just as fair to label insulin the "energy hormone," or the "sugar transport hormone." Insulin becomes a fat storage hormone only after it has met our current energy needs *and* has filled up our glycogen reserves to the best of its ability. Furthermore, insulin will not cause fat gain in the absence of positive energy balance, a point we went over in Chapter 1.

Now, if you like, go ahead and pick up your favorite low carbohydrate diet book, and refer to that for a description of insulin's fat-promoting effects. Insulin-bashing is mainstream in the diet industry. Everyone is doing it. However, we have already discussed the problem with the "insulin makes you fat" model. That problem being that the latest dietary research disproves many of the claims that proponents of low carbohydrate diets make. If you would like to frame your diet in terms of "insulin makes you fat," then you bolster my argument that caffeine contributes to weight gain, because it is well settled that caffeine raises blood sugar and insulin levels, and also contributes to insulin resistance.[128]

Since caffeine raises insulin and blood sugar levels, it would be convenient for me to adopt the "insulin makes you fat" framework in this chapter, but that would be intellectually incomplete and perhaps dishonest given the latest research on the subject. I do propose that high levels of insulin are a problem for the dieter, but that this is due to insulin's promotion of overeating, and therefore insulin's contribution to positive energy balance, rather than any supposed intrinsic fat-promoting insulin mechanism.

The problem that insulin presents for weight loss is that large amounts of this hormone can cause problems with blood sugar regulation, which lead to uncontrollable cravings and an inability to feel full. The first way in which insulin contributes to overeating is through insulin resistance, and the second way is through hypoglycemia. We will discuss these problems in turn.

The Resistance

With the abuse of starches, sugars, and caffeine that is prevalent in modern diets, insulin becomes less and less efficient at its task of delivering blood glucose to the cells that need it.[129] This creates a condition called insulin resistance, which means that a normal amount of insulin is no longer enough to meet the body's glucose transport needs. In insulin resistance, the body does not use insulin efficiently, so the pancreas is forced to produce more insulin in order to keep your blood glucose under control. An insulin resistant individual may produce up to five times as much insulin as a non-insulin resistant individual in response to the same amount of carbohydrate.[130]

Insulin resistance is associated with a number of health problems, especially weight gain and obesity. In insulin resistance, the body's muscle, fat, and liver cells do not respond properly to insulin's efforts to make these cells accept glucose. Since glucose is not being accepted by the body's cells, it remains at an elevated level in the blood. Insulin-producing cells in the pancreas continue to respond to the elevated blood glucose by producing more insulin, and finally, after a time, the higher insulin levels are able to get the glucose to where it needs to be.

Insulin resistance is self perpetuating. The more insulin that is produced by the body, the more desensitized the body's cells become to insulin, and the more desensitized the cells become to insulin, the more insulin the body produces to try to get these cells to accept glucose. At the cellular level, high levels of insulin in the body contribute to insulin resistance by gradually desensitizing the body's cells to insulin's action.[131]

This means that it is a chronically elevated insulin level itself that causes insulin resistance to develop over time. Furthermore, and significantly for our purposes, the overproduction of insulin that is produced in the insulin resistant individual can result in blood sugar and insulin fluctuations that perpetuate hunger and overeating, especially of sugar and starch, which further exacerbate the condition.

Insulin resistance can be thought of as a high level of insulin in the body, resulting in, among other symptoms, increased appetite and overeating. Hunger is one of the most common symptoms of insulin resistance, and those individuals who experience this symptom relieve it by overeating. Insulin resistance brings on strong feelings of hunger because the body's cells are not receiving energy, and are literally starving to be fed.

Due to the inability of insulin to efficiently feed glucose to the body's cells, sufferers of insulin resistance find themselves constantly hungry. Insulin resistance also causes hunger because high levels of insulin destabilize blood sugar, causing blood sugar to drop, and low blood sugar makes us hungry, as we'll discuss in some depth in a moment.

Insulin resistance can become type 2 diabetes later in life, when the supply of insulin from the pancreas finally runs out. Type 2 diabetes runs in some families, so if members of your family have had this disease, you are at a greater risk of developing it yourself. Without insulin from the pancreas to regulate blood sugar levels, blood sugar can become dangerously high and can cause damage to all of the body's organs. High blood glucose levels are especially dangerous to the heart, blood vessels, liver, kidneys, and eyes. This is the reason that type 2 diabetes often leads to death from heart disease, as blood vessels and the heart become damaged by high levels of circulating blood sugar.

In a study that followed 276 individuals for six years, researchers discovered that insulin secretion in response to food intake predicted weight gain.[132] The more insulin that an individual produced in response to food intake, the more weight that individual gained over the period of the study. Furthermore, the researchers noted that for some individuals who produce more insulin than average, these individuals gain a lot of weight on a diet that is high in carbohydrates, suggesting that a genetic or environmental factor may be involved.[133]

In other words, some individuals are prone to overproduce insulin, for any one of a number of reasons, and gain more weight on diets that provoke high levels of insulin production. This weight gain is likely due to insulin-induced hunger and overeating. Moreover, individuals who overproduce insulin due to genetic factors would feel hungrier and be more prone to overeating than the average person due to the insulin-spiking effects of caffeine. The more sensitive your insulin system is to carbohydrate, the more sensitive your insulin system will be to caffeine, because caffeine consumption provokes the same blood glucose and insulin responses that carbohydrate does, even if the caffeine is taken without added sugar or a pastry.

Some nutrition writers insist that insulin resistance itself is the cause of weight gain, rather than a symptom of the broader problem of overeating. When we overeat, we increase our energy intake and also increase our insulin levels, assuming that part of our energy intake comes from protein or carbohydrates, both of which increase insulin levels.

If overeating leads to weight gain and insulin resistance, the causative agent here is overeating, not insulin resistance. As we discussed in Chapter 1, energy balance, rather than hormonal balance, is the key to weight loss, and hormonal balance is only relevant to the extent that it helps us maintain our desired level of energy balance to achieve our weight loss goals. But in any event, a large portion of the nutrition writers currently tell us that insulin resistance contributes to weight gain by mechanisms other than insulin-induced hunger and overeating.

I contend that it is insulin-induced hunger and overeating due to insulin resistance-starved cells and unsteady blood sugar levels that cause the weight gain blamed on insulin. It is not insulin by itself, but the contribution of high levels of insulin to our overeating behavior.

Caffeine

In lean, healthy individuals, caffeine raises blood sugar and insulin levels.[134] Caffeine intake reduces the insulin sensitivity of muscle cells, so that the muscle cells can not accept glucose at a normal rate, which results in blood glucose and insulin levels remaining elevated. Muscle is the major tissue that becomes insulin resistant after caffeine ingestion, so that glucose can not enter muscle the way it normally can when the body is not exposed to caffeine.

Studies have confirmed that caffeine consumption reduces the whole body's ability to use glucose by 15-30%, and glucose use in the leg muscle by approximately 50%.[135] By closing off the body's cells to glucose, caffeine causes the body's tissues to be exposed to insulin for longer periods of time than they would be in the absence of caffeine consumption. By creating this insulin resistant state, caffeine ingestion creates elevated insulin levels in the blood, and contributes to the development of caffeine-independent insulin resistance and type 2 diabetes over time. Furthermore, caffeine ingestion disrupts the body's glucose and insulin systems to an even greater degree when it is taken in conjunction with sugar and other carbohydrates, creating an additive effect and further spiking insulin levels.

The stress response to caffeine ingestion also has an influence on our blood sugar levels. When we experience stress, the stress hormones cortisol and epinephrine cause a release of glucose from stored glycogen throughout our body, which elevates blood sugar levels and brings about a corresponding increase in insulin to regulate the now raised blood sugar. Cortisol can raise blood sugar levels all by itself, and this explains in part how caffeine causes insulin and blood sugar levels to rise even if it is taken without sugar.

The other part of the explanation is caffeine's insulin-de-sensitizing effect on muscle cells, through which it closes off these muscle cells to glucose and thereby prompts the body to produce more insulin to deal with the stubborn, high blood sugar level. The body's glucose and insulin responses to caffeine are very interesting. Caffeine makes the body's cells spit out their stored glucose into the blood, while disabling muscle cells from taking this glucose back up as glycogen, prompting insulin levels to increase further and further until the insulin can finally convince the body's cells to accept enough glucose to bring blood sugar levels down to a desirable level.

Caffeine contributes to the development of insulin resistance, pre-diabetes (a condition just short of type 2 diabetes characterized by high blood sugar), and type 2 diabetes over time. Risk factors for the development of insulin resistance and pre-diabetes include: being physically inactive, having a parent or sibling with diabetes, having a family background that is African American, Alaska Native, American Indian, Asian American, Hispanic/Latino, or Pacific Islander, giving birth to a baby weighing more than 9 pounds or being diagnosed with gestational diabetes, having high blood pressure (140/90 or above), having an HDL (good cholesterol) level below 35 mg/dL or a triglyceride level above 250 mg/dL, having polycystic ovary syndrome (PCOS), having impaired fasting glucose (IFG) or impaired glucose tolerance (IGT), severe obesity, or a history of cardiovascular disease.

Signs and symptoms that are associated with insulin resistance (and also overeating) include weight gain and difficulty losing weight (especially visceral adiposity, which is belly fat underneath the abdominal muscle wall), fatigue, difficulty in concentrating, intestinal bloating, high blood sugar, sleepiness (especially after eating), elevated triglycerides, elevated blood pressure, and depression. Judging by these symptoms, it might be safe to give a preliminary diagnosis of insulin resistance to most Americans. A sedentary lifestyle and elevated cortisol levels are also associated with insulin resistance.

In the previous chapter we discussed how chronically elevated cortisol levels relocate fat stores to deep within the abdominal wall. This accumulation of visceral fat also negatively affects the insulin sensitivity of our body's cells, further contributes to insulin resistance, and is a strong predictor of type 2 diabetes.[136] There are strong links between insulin resistance and visceral fat, as distinct from subcutaneous fat.

Subcutaneous fat is fat between the skin and muscle wall, and is the kind of fat that we can pinch. Visceral fat, on the other hand, is the fat that surrounds our internal organs and that we are unable to pinch or poke with our fingers. Visceral fat produces proteins called cytokines, which have been found to alter normal insulin activity throughout the body, contributing to insulin resistance.

This is another way in which insulin resistance perpetuates itself, by setting an individual up for weight gain through increased hunger, and part of this weight gain will be visceral fat, which will further promote problems with insulin. Visceral adiposity is also correlated with an increase of fat in the liver, known as fatty liver disease.

Fatty liver disease is the most common liver disease in America, presenting itself as a large amount of fat in the liver cells. The result of fatty liver disease is a large amount of free fatty acids being released into the bloodstream and an increase of glucose production which, you guessed it, further aggravate insulin resistance.

An easy test for insulin resistance risk that you can do at home and that is both fairly reliable and cheap is the waist circumference test. Take a measuring tape and take your waist measurement at the level of your belly button. If you are a man and the tape measures your waist at over 40 inches, then you are at risk for, and may already have insulin resistance. If you are a woman and the tape measures your waist at over 35 inches, then you are at risk for, and may already have insulin resistance.

This is not a perfect tool, as there are thin individuals who are insulin resistant and overweight individuals who are not insulin resistant, but this measurement is nevertheless useful. If your waist measurement puts you at risk, you should give your insulin levels some thought so as to avoid type 2 diabetes and cardiovascular disease in the future.

The overproduction of insulin in our bodies is a widespread problem that goes beyond weight gain, with severe long-term health consequences. Perhaps this is why nutrition writers exaggerate insulin's role in fat gain, in order to wake people up to the importance of cutting back on refined carbohydrates.

What are our weapons in the battle to keep our insulin levels under control? First, low carbohydrate diets have been shown to help in reducing insulin resistance.[137] In addition to a reduced carbohydrate diet, reducing our caffeine consumption will also help by removing caffeine-induced insulin resistance and the caffeine-induced blood glucose and insulin spikes.

Next, physical activity and weight loss help improve the body's response to insulin, thereby reducing insulin resistance. Specifically, exercise helps to reverse the insulin resistance of muscle cells, allowing these cells to improve their ability to take in glucose quickly and efficiently.[138] In this way, exercise has the opposite effect of caffeine on muscle cells. While caffeine closes these cells off to the receipt of glucose, exercise helps to open them again. Muscle is the main site of glucose disposal in the body, so its ready acceptance of glucose is critically important in maintaining steady, healthy blood glucose and insulin levels.[139] We will address exercise in Chapter 7, the Decaf Plan.

In addition to physical activity and weight loss, a higher intake of vitamin D may also help to combat insulin resistance, as vitamin D deficiency is associated with insulin resistance.[140] To improve your vitamin D status, you should strive to expose your body to the sun's rays for short periods of time on a regular basis.

Finally, and I include this as a note rather than as a recommendation, intermittent fasting improves insulin's ability to bring glucose to the body's cells.[141] What is interesting here is that it is the fasting that helps improve insulin sensitivity, rather than a reduction in food intake or any changes in macronutrient balance. The study participants who fasted continued to eat the same diet and in the same quantity, but they shifted their eating to make it more concentrated at certain times, while having no food at other times. This scheduling change was enough to improve the body's insulin sensitivity in the study, perhaps because it mimicked the eating pattern on which our bodies evolved, that of alternating periods of feast and famine.

Does this mean that if we exercise, get adequate sunshine, and reduce our carbohydrate intake, that caffeine will no longer be able to produce an insulin resistant state in our bodies? This is exactly what one group of researchers sought to discover: whether periods of insulin resistance brought about by caffeine consumption would be reduced or eliminated if individuals lost weight and adopted a healthier diet.[142]

The researchers discovered that weight loss and aerobic exercise did *not* reduce caffeine's ability to bring about an insulin resistant state in the body, even though weight loss and exercise are effective strategies for non-caffeine-induced insulin resistance. In other words, while you want to increase your body's insulin sensitivity in general, the steps you take will not prevent the insulin desensitizing effect of caffeine on your muscle cells. That being said, improving your body's insulin sensitivity will make your body able to deal with caffeine-induced insulin resistance more rapidly, and if your insulin system is healthy, the effects of caffeine-induced insulin resistance will be mitigated.

Low Blood Sugar

Now that we have a handle on caffeine-induced insulin resistance and the elevated blood glucose and insulin levels that result, let's examine the related problem of low blood sugar. The phenomenon of low blood sugar levels in response to food intake is called reactive hypoglycemia. Hypoglycemia is the medical term for low blood sugar, and reactive hypoglycemia is the low blood sugar that results in reaction to food or drink that provokes a large insulin response.

Insulin resistance and hypoglycemia are both indicative of an overproduction of insulin in the body, and sometimes present themselves simultaneously. The overproduction of insulin in insulin resistance can lead to hypoglycemia, which then leads to carbohydrate cravings, which further exacerbate insulin resistance and destabilize blood sugar levels, and so forth, in a self-perpetuating cycle. This is why feeding cravings for sugar and starch usually just ensures that these cravings come back soon after.

Caffeine can produce reactive hypoglycemia by its over-stimulation of insulin, which in some people will bring blood glucose levels below their normal range. Moderate amounts of caffeine can bring about a hypoglycemic state in the body just as ingesting a large amount of carbohydrates can.[143] The hypoglycemic effects of caffeine consumption are well understood, (the drop in blood sugar is the aftereffect of a caffeine-induced spike in blood glucose and insulin levels) but it is still somewhat unclear why some individuals are more sensitive to these effects than others. This is explained by individual differences (biochemical individuality) in the health of our insulin systems due to genetic, environmental, nutritional, and lifestyle factors.

Caffeine-induced low blood sugar can lead to uncontrollable cravings for carbohydrate-rich foods, and in this way lead to overeating. Hypoglycemia often results in biologically driven cravings that are next to impossible to resist, and the avoidance of low blood sugar is another reason that low carbohydrate diets often succeed in producing high levels of satiety. Hypoglycemia is sometimes a precursor to type 2 diabetes, especially when it is not controlled with diet. If you are a hypoglycemic, your main concern should be to prevent your blood sugar from spiking and dropping, and caffeine is one of the low blood sugar villains you must avoid.

Hypoglycemia is often the result of a diet high in sugar, alcohol, and caffeine. The symptoms of hypoglycemia include intense and sudden hunger, cravings for sweets, dizziness, weakness, fatigue, sweating, cold hands and feet, mental confusion, mood swings, nervousness, trembling, heart palpitations, insomnia and trouble speaking. For many hypoglycemics, a strong cup of coffee can bring on a number of these symptoms. Hypoglycemia brings with it an urgency to eat and a resolution of symptoms once food is taken. This is how insulin can be a strong driver of overeating for those people who experience the symptoms of low blood sugar.

Due to genetic variation, some people have higher baseline levels of insulin than others, and as a result, these overproducers of insulin are more likely to have problems both with low blood sugar and with insulin resistance. This explains why some people are more susceptible to reactive hypoglycemia and rebound overeating than others. When your blood sugar gets too low due to an overproduction of insulin, you may experience rebound overeating as your body tries to bring your glucose levels back up via food intake.

This is why stable blood sugar levels are so important for weight loss and the maintenance of a lean physique, because stable blood sugar levels promote satiety. For people who are prone to low blood sugar episodes, steady blood sugar means a controlled appetite, and a controlled appetite means a reduced food intake.

I have experienced rebound overeating myself, as I suffered with hypoglycemia for a time and to this day I am sometimes haunted by this condition. My hypoglycemia started, as health problems often do, when I was a stressed graduate student preparing for finals. My diet consisted mostly of sandwiches which I made for myself and, you guessed it, copious amounts of coffee. I would hurry to make myself a couple of turkey sandwiches, rush to the library, and fill my coffee mug.

I felt very fortunate at the time to be living in a library that had its own café. My coffee mug was never empty, and after some time on this regime, I began to experience extreme dizziness and weakness. I did not have any of the other symptoms aside from an increased urgency to eat, even though I was not actually hungry when this feeling came. The shakiness I felt was almost unbearable, I sometimes felt so dizzy that it was difficult for me walk straight, and I felt that if I did not eat something sweet and starchy immediately, I would keel over and die.

I tried to figure out what the problem was, and had some blood work done. My blood sugar was low, but not low enough that alarm bells went off for the doctor. I looked up the condition of low blood sugar, discovered that coffee aggravated this condition, and stopped drinking coffee. My symptoms resolved themselves immediately, and I felt fine again.

But to this day, I can reproduce my extreme dizziness by consuming two standard cups of coffee in a short period of time, and caffeine affects me much more so than do carbohydrates in producing symptoms of hypoglycemia. The effect is even greater, however, when I put sugar in the coffee or consume other carbohydrates close in time with my coffee drinking. Fortunately, low blood sugar is taken more seriously these days than it was previously, so it is much easier to become educated about this condition and work to resolve it.

Let's go over what was happening inside my body during these hypoglycemic episodes. The coffee that I was drinking, even though I was usually taking it without sugar, was raising my blood glucose levels and making my muscle cells insulin resistant, and thereby raising my insulin levels. My insulin levels were being raised high enough that they would decrease my blood sugar levels to such a low level as to make me feel the unpleasant symptoms of hypoglycemia, and these symptoms would drive me to eat sugary, calorie-laden foods to relieve my symptoms. Once I had taken this food, my blood sugar levels would rise again and over time the insulin and glucose would strike a balance, at least until I had my next cup of coffee.

Sometimes I would let the dizziness and shakiness go on and resolve on its own, and it usually did so within an hour or two, but I sometimes felt the effects for longer periods of time, even through the end of the day. The stress I was under at the time no doubt contributed to the effects I was feeling, and I am sometimes able to consume caffeine without the dizziness and shakiness accompanying my caffeine consumption, if I have the caffeine-containing beverage on its own and in low amounts. Now, many years later, I know after reading through other people's experiences with hypoglycemia, that coffee can be one of the worst offenders for sufferers of this condition.

Whether or not you have symptoms of hypoglycemia, you can be sure that caffeine is raising your insulin levels and increasing your chances of developing insulin resistance in the long run. In turn, insulin resistance increases the chances of developing type 2 diabetes and heart disease. Insulin resistance also goes hand in hand with pre-diabetes, a condition in which blood glucose levels are higher than normal but not high enough for a diagnosis of full diabetes.

Both insulin resistance and pre-diabetes are relatively asymptomatic, so a person may have one or both of these conditions for years without being aware of them. As we've already noted, caffeine worsens insulin resistance and pre-diabetic conditions all by itself, even if the caffeine-containing beverage is taken without sugar.

Armed with this observation, researchers have noted that individuals trying to lose weight and control blood sugar who are suffering from insulin resistance or pre-diabetes should decrease or eliminate dietary caffeine. Along with a reduction of caffeine, increased exercise and an improved diet have been found to be the most effective means of correcting blood sugar and insulin problems.[144] As for using exercise to help address the problem of insulin resistance, researchers have even discovered that it is carbohydrate deficit after exercise, rather than total energy deficit, that contributes to an increase in insulin sensitivity, lending further support to the importance of carbohydrate control for a healthy insulin system.[145]

A reduction of your caffeine intake will reduce the resultant caffeine-induced glucose and insulin spikes. Should you choose to retain some or all of your caffeine consumption, however, you should try to have your caffeine separately from other foods that are loaded with carbohydrates, as carbohydrate-rich foods taken in conjunction with caffeine will make the caffeine-induced hunger and overeating worse. This is one way of improving your caffeine consumption without quitting, and this method and others will be reviewed in the upcoming chapters, The Decaf Plan and Optimal Caffeine Use.

Evil Hormones?

Although we will revisit cortisol briefly in the chapter, Diet Pills, Green Tea, and the Thyroid, since we have finished most of our discussion about insulin and cortisol, let's think about why these hormones do what they do. Why do these two vital hormones make us overeat? We need both cortisol and insulin in healthy amounts to survive, so what gives? From an evolutionary perspective, it makes sense that these hormones cause us to overeat.

Let's start with cortisol. Cortisol encourages us to overeat in times of stress, and when that stress was running away from a deadly predator, overeating afterwards would replace the energy we lost in the chase, and also refuel us for our next escape. In addition, the relocation of fat stores to the center of the body would make that energy easiest to mobilize when we encountered the next deadly predator and had to run again. The relocation of fat stores to the center of our bodies would also create some cushion for our internal organs which could be harmed during our getaway.

As for insulin, this hormone helped the human species to put on fat when food was plentiful, in preparation for famine and for winter. A little insulin-resistance-induced overeating is healthy when it helps us to put on the fat we need to survive a coming winter, when food will be scarce. That vitamin D increases insulin sensitivity helps lend support to the theory of seasonal weight gain being a part of our evolutionary past. Less vitamin D means more insulin resistance, and more insulin resistance means more overeating due to insulin-induced hunger.

Decreasing amounts of sunlight and the corresponding decreasing amounts of vitamin D in our blood would have signaled a coming winter, and the ability to develop insulin resistance in response to low vitamin D and overeat when this environmental cue presents itself would have been a favorable survival trait in climates with cold winters. Today, when food is plentiful year-round, we no longer need the ability to shift to "winter metabolism."

In controlled amounts, both of these hormones are necessary for our survival, but when they become chronically elevated, their effects on hunger make overeating difficult to avoid. When food was scarce and predators roamed freely, we needed these hormones to help us consume and store as much energy as possible, but now that we live in a society where food is in abundance and hungry stalking predators are rare, the same hormones that have kept us alive throughout the centuries are now making us fat.

The ability to become insulin resistant helped us to over-eat for short periods of time in order to put on the fat that would power our bodies during lean times when food was unavailable. But there are no longer any lean times, at least not in the modern day United States. Similarly, cortisol-induced overeating was a boon when we faced intense in-termittent stressors, and now that those intermittent stres-sors have become one constant stressor of caffeine con-sumption, lack of sleep and a hectic life, cortisol now runs free, to our detriment.

Now that we are heavy users of caffeine, cortisol and insu-lin levels are chronically elevated. In effect, caffeine gives these two hormones free reign to encourage us to overeat constantly, even though we live in a society of plenty and do not need to store large amounts of fat to survive. Part of the problem is that we have not had a large enough amount of time to adapt to the presence of caffeine in our diets, and to the presence of so much food in our lives, so we have found ourselves at a disadvantage because of the health and aes-thetic problems that year-round fat gain presents.

If you go through one or both of the plans at the end of this book for caffeine reduction and optimal caffeine use, you will be going a long way to getting your insulin and corti-sol levels back under control, and in so doing you will sig-nificantly decrease your overeating behavior, and become leaner, meaner, and healthier.

Summary

Caffeine raises your body's blood glucose and insulin lev-els. Caffeine also directly creates an insulin resistant state in the body after it is consumed. The elevations in glucose and insulin brought about by caffeine exacerbate insulin resistance and problems with blood sugar regulation. The result is hunger and cravings for carbohydrate-rich foods because the body's cells are being starved by insulin resistance and because of low blood sugar spells. This insulin-induced hunger leads to overeating, which contributes to positive energy balance, making weight loss and maintenance of a lean physique difficult.

Maintaining steady, healthy levels of blood glucose and insulin is one of the keys to lasting satiety and a controlled appetite. Ways to improve blood sugar and insulin regulation include caffeine reduction, a restriction of carbohydrate taken with caffeine-containing foods and beverages, carbohydrate restriction generally, exercise, weight loss, exposure to sunlight, and intermittent fasting. In Chapter 8, Optimal Caffeine Use, we will fully discuss how you can continue to consume caffeine while blunting the negative effects of this drug for your blood sugar and insulin levels. In the next chapter, we will discuss some more distinct ways in which caffeine causes overeating.

CHAPTER 5
ADDICTION-DRIVEN OVEREATING

*Only Irish coffee provides in a single glass all four
essential food groups: alcohol, caffeine, sugar, and fat.*
                                                    -Alex Levine

Without sounding too much like conspiracy theorists, let's admit that the goal of the caffeine industry is to get you hooked on their products. Whether it's coffee, tea, soda, energy drinks, or any other caffeine-containing product, peddling addictive products is excellent business. Caffeine not only gives us a bit of a mood lift when we consume it, but it also makes us feel horrible when we stop consuming it, and these two properties of caffeine make it a bestseller.

Like oil, coffee is one of the most valuable export commodities on the planet.[146] Once we are addicted to caffeine, we have to keep coming back to our caffeinated product of choice in order to stave off the unpleasant withdrawal symptoms. Furthermore, caffeine, once consumed, is gone, so we are forced to keep making donations to our favorite caffeine sellers to get more. For the seller, an addictive product is a perfect one.

And that's a good segue for talking about *Dune*, Frank Herbert's 1965 science fiction classic. The plot of *Dune* involves a violent struggle between opposing forces to gain control of the desert planet Arrakis, which is the only known source of the spice "melange," the most valuable substance in the universe. The spice of Arrakis is commonly interpreted as a metaphor for oil; however, I think it is more convincing as a metaphor for caffeine.

Melange is a drug that gives its users greater vitality, increased awareness, and in some cases prescience, allowing for safer interstellar travel. This parallels the increase in mental alertness and wakefulness that caffeine provides for its users, as well as a corresponding ability to compose boring research papers and to stay awake on the road for many hours.

The melange of *Dune* is addictive, and withdrawal is fatal. Caffeine is also addictive, and though withdrawal is not fatal, it can sometimes feel that way. Melange is the most important substance in the universe in *Dune*, and it is similar in some ways to caffeine. There have been many violent struggles behind the scenes of coffee production, and most of us are unfamiliar with the violence in coffee-producing nations over this valuable commodity. If you would like to learn more, *Uncommon Grounds,* by Mark Pendergrast, is a good starting point. Perhaps Herbert was even predicting a future in which coffee overtakes oil as the most valuable export commodity on our planet. If we stop or modify our usage of fossil fuels, that scenario may well play out.

In addition to the implications of Frank Herbert's *Dune,* this chapter considers the consumption of foods and nutrients that are taken in conjunction with caffeine. By most accounts, caffeine is an addictive substance, and once we are addicted to it, we can not resist consuming it, and with it, all the sugar and fat that accompanies the particular caffeinated product of our choosing. This is one more way in which caffeine contributes to overeating and weight gain.

An Acquired Taste

Most people don't like the taste of coffee the first time they try it, finding it bitter and even unpalatable. After trying it a few times, however, most of us become accustomed to the taste and develop a liking for the stuff. Why is coffee an acquired taste? Research suggests that we develop a preference for those tastes, flavors, and aromas that we associate with the effects of a drug, in this case caffeine, through conditioning.[147] In other words, the effects of the drug program us to enjoy the foods and beverages that contain it.

So although we don't actually like the taste of coffee at first, once we have experienced the effects of the drug caffeine via coffee, we associate the two, and we acquire the taste for coffee, because we like the stimulation. The fictional drug melange, too, is an acquired taste, its drug content encouraging the body to learn to find its flavor pleasurable.[148] In the case of sodas or chocolate candy, there is no learning period to go through because the sweetness of these foods makes them instant hits.

Addiction

Caffeine is an addictive drug. The three criteria used for evaluating the addictiveness of a substance are psychoactivity, substance dependence, and reinforcing effects.[149] As to the first criterion, the determination of whether a drug is psychoactive is made by looking at its effects on mood and behavior. Since a wide range of studies have confirmed that caffeine improves mood at low levels of consumption and increases anxiety at higher levels of consumption, researchers have determined that caffeine is a psychoactive drug, having effects on mood and behavior with which most of us are familiar.[150]

As to substance dependence, an examination of this criterion focuses on the development of tolerance, withdrawal, the inability to stop using the substance, and continued use over a long period of time.[151] A study on caffeine tolerance indicates that 75% of the participants who used low amounts of caffeine relative to the national average developed a tolerance, leading to a need for higher doses of caffeine in order to maintain the same physiological effects.[152]

As we have seen, however, caffeine's effects on the body's stress levels do not decrease with continual use. There is no corresponding tolerance developed to caffeine's effect of raising our cortisol levels. We develop a tolerance in that we experience less of caffeine's pleasant effects over time, but not less of caffeine's negative effects. Not nice.

Most individuals (over 90% in one study) experience withdrawal symptoms upon the discontinuation of caffeine use that include insomnia, loss of coordination, headaches, tension, fatigue, decreased attention, increased anxiety, irritability, nausea and vomiting, depression, bad mood, and increased heart rates.[153] The existence of these withdrawal symptoms lends support to the conclusion that caffeine is addictive.

Even if you are only consuming the caffeine equivalent of one cup of coffee per day (100 mg), you are likely to experience some withdrawal symptoms. This is a low daily caffeine intake by conventional standards, and yet this low intake is sufficient to produce some of the unpleasant withdrawal symptoms described above.

Some caffeine researchers have found that it is exactly these withdrawal symptoms that keep us coming back; giving us the illusion that caffeine makes us feel good when in reality it is only helping us to not feel the ill effects of missing our fix. This is called the withdrawal reversal or withdrawal alleviation model of caffeine consumption.

In effect, habitual caffeine consumers self-administer the drug in order to alleviate their withdrawal symptoms... from the drug itself.[154] The researchers testing this model of caffeine consumption discovered that individuals who experienced withdrawal symptoms were more likely to take caffeine than those individuals who experienced no symptoms. Another study suggests that the only benefit of caffeine use is its removal of withdrawal symptoms, and that there is no overall benefit because by removing the withdrawal symptoms, caffeine merely restores our performance and feelings of well-being to normal levels.[155]

Withdrawal symptoms can arise within hours of missing a regular dose of caffeine, and the relief of these symptoms through caffeine consumption contributes to the maintenance of our caffeine habit.[156] The fast onset of unpleasantness after missing our regular cup of coffee or tea forces many of us to keep caffeine close at hand and a regular part of our lives. Devious.

Most habitual caffeine consumers also have difficulties with stopping caffeine consumption even in the face of problems resulting from the drug's continued use, leading researchers to conclude that caffeine dependence should be recognized as a clinical syndrome.[157] As to the continued use of caffeine over a long period of time, this is something with which we are all familiar.

We don't need a study that demonstrates that most people consume caffeine for their whole lives; we are those people.

Finally, caffeine has been found to have reinforcing properties, as its consumption provides both stimulation and
relief to the user, and its use begets further use.[158] Reinforcing effects can best be described as an individual's craving
for a drug that increases with use of the drug, so the more
you take, the more you want.

Given the preceding discussion, it is clear that caffeine neat-
ly fits the technical definition of an addictive substance. At
least as important as caffeine's technical designation as an
addictive substance is the way most caffeine consumers actually act and feel in relation to this drug. The withdrawal
symptoms that come with stopping caffeine intake and the
difficulty most people have in abstaining from caffeine say
enough about caffeine's addictive impact on its consumers.
Most people, outside of the above studies and in real life,
are hooked on caffeine and can not get off of this drug.

In my own experience, caffeine slowly crept into my life
and I found myself gradually increasing the amount of caffeine I consumed both to alleviate the withdrawal symptoms and to maintain the positive effects I experienced
from caffeine. Before long, I wasn't just drinking coffee at
work to get myself through an assignment; I was drinking
coffee on the weekends and on vacations. I began to rely on
the stuff, just as many of us do. Over time, however, I found
that I consumed more and more caffeine but was not getting any pleasant feelings from my coffee or tea anymore; it
was only helping to stave off the headaches and fatigue that
came when I missed one of my regular doses.

Along with the caffeine that had entered my life, so had the
sugar and fat in my coffee, tea, and chocolate. These calories had not been in my life before, and even apart from the
hormonal effects of caffeine, the influx of calories that is
usually a part of caffeine-containing foods and beverages is
enough, by itself, to cause weight gain.

93

Side Calories

The presence of side calories in caffeinated foods and beverages is another way that caffeine consumption leads to overeating, and contributes to positive energy balance. Along with the caffeine that we receive from the cup of coffee necessary to satisfy our habit, we get side calories in the drink in the form of cream, sugar, milk, and whatever else we put in the coffee.

With the success of Starbucks and its new vocabulary of beverages, we are now confronted by some very calorie-dense coffee. Additionally, if, out of force of habit, we are used to eating a pastry with our morning cup such that it is part of the coffee ritual, then we consume these side calories as part of our caffeine habit as well.

Starbucks makes some of the most popular caffeinated beverages on the market. And these caffeinated beverages often exceed 200 calories per serving, and sometimes contain over 500 calories. That's a liquid meal. Starbucks is not alone in packing its caffeinated drinks with large amounts of calories. Many other coffee, energy drink, and iced tea companies do it too. A 16 ounce bottle of Snapple iced tea, for example, has about 180 calories, all from sugar. Of course as we are all becoming more health conscious, these companies have met our demand for lower calorie caffeinated beverages, and we have more and more options in the market to reduce our consumption of side calories along with caffeine.

It is these side calories that further exacerbate caffeine's impact on the over-consumption of calories. Is this to say we should drink our tea and coffee without cream and sugar? That is a step in the right direction, and we'll return to that in the chapter entitled, Optimal Caffeine Use. A small shift in calories, cutting just the cream or sugar or both from your coffee, can have a very large impact on your body composition over time.

Chocoholics Anonymous

What if you are eating chocolate for the caffeine? You're in trouble! A large amount of side calories is usually found in chocolate-containing foods since we prefer to take our chocolate in candy, cookie, cake, or ice cream form. Our desire to consume chocolate and chocolate-containing foods is driven both by caffeine and theobromine. Although caffeine is present in relatively small amounts in chocolate when compared to coffee and tea, chocolate is the main source of theobromine in the human diet.

Some believe that theobromine is as addictive as caffeine, or at least similarly addictive. Although hard evidence is still somewhat lacking on the topic of chocolate's addictive characteristics, there is ample anecdotal evidence to support a conclusion that chocolate is habit-forming. A large number of self-professed "chocoholics" claim that they can not quit the substance, and given that chocolate-containing foods usually have a large amount of side calories, the implications of "chocolate addiction" for weight gain are worthy of consideration.

I must admit that I am a recovering chocoholic. There are many chocoholics out there, some recovering, some active, and some in between. Some consume chocolate on a daily basis, but for others several times weekly is sufficient to satisfy their cravings. When I fall off the wagon, I fall into the first category – that of needing some chocolate almost every day. I'm not sure why I'm vulnerable to this habit given that it usually affects women more severely than men, but perhaps it is genetic.

My father is a chocoholic, and he loves dark chocolate, the really dark stuff. Perhaps I inherited my chocolate habit from him (my mother can take it or leave it). These days I am able to keep this habit under control by limiting my overall sugar intake, and I'll explain what that's about in the Fructose and Sugar Addiction sections coming up in this chapter. When I do consume chocolate, I do so in accordance with the rules in Chapter 8, Optimal Caffeine Use.

Origins of chocoholism aside, regular chocoholics and occasional chocoholics such as myself face a huge problem. Just about all of the chocolate on the market comes in a high calorie package. A 100 gram bar of dark chocolate, for example, typically contains about 500 calories. These calories are mainly from the fat in the form of cocoa butter and the added sugars in the chocolate. Other chocolate products are also calorie-dense. Chocolate ice cream, chocolate cookies, and chocolate cake are prominent examples. We don't need to go through the per serving nutritional information for each of these items to know that these items are extremely calorie-dense. And most of us mere mortals cannot restrict ourselves to one serving anyway.

People who crave and consume chocolate, therefore, get much more than they bargain for if all their bodies crave is the theobromine fix or the particular combination of theobromine and caffeine found in chocolate. In the upcoming chapter on optimal caffeine consumption, I will describe how you can satisfy your chocolate cravings while drastically cutting the side calories that chocolate products contain. I also describe a similar strategy for all caffeine products should you choose to keep these products in your diet.

Chocolate contains flavanols that have been found to have some benefits, including increased blood flow to the brain, and chocolate producers desperately latch on to any positive chocolate studies to promote their products. It's fashionable these days to say that chocolate is healthy, proving that advertising works. And while I am not saying that there is no benefit whatsoever from the plant compounds in chocolate, I am saying that these benefits may be significantly outweighed (pun intended) by chocolate's fat-promoting effects.

Perhaps the chocolatey boost in blood flow to the brain is strong enough to counteract the decreased blood flow from caffeine's blood vessel-constricting effects, perhaps not. The study that found a brain-boosting effect of chocolate used a specially formulated cocoa beverage that provides levels of flavanols unavailable in any commercially available cocoa or chocolate product.[159] Go figure. Flavanols are not unique to chocolate, of course, and can be found in a variety of fruits and vegetables; berries and red wine are popular sources. Fruits and vegetables can replace any possible benefits of caffeinated foods and beverages, especially the supposed benefits of calorie-dense chocolate products.

Big Kids

The effects of caffeine on young children have not been studied extensively, and this alarms some groups because of children's preferences for soft drinks and the successful marketing of these caffeine-laden beverages to children.[160] The studies that have been done on children demonstrate that children respond to caffeine as they would to an addictive substance, displaying both withdrawal symptoms when caffeine is discontinued and the reinforcing effects of caffeine use.[161] Children are often the target of soft drink advertising, and from a business point of view this makes a lot of sense. The sooner that soda companies can hook a child on caffeine, the sooner he will become a lifelong customer. For children, the high sugar content of soft drinks makes these beverages the perfect delivery system for caffeine. Not only do soft drinks provide the sugar kids love, but the sugar also effectively masks the bitter caffeine that will keep those kids coming back for more.

For years, soft drinks have been gaining momentum as a fixture in schools throughout the world. This caught the attention of a number of consumer advocacy groups, including the World Heart Federation, which is trying to get sugary beverages out of schools around the world as part of its fight against childhood obesity. In 2006, PepsiCo adopted guidelines to remove its sugary soft drinks from schools around the world by 2012, replacing these beverages with water, milk, and juice without added sugar.

Coca-Cola has been more reluctant to give in to the World Heart Federation's global demands, but has agreed to stay out of elementary schools unless the parents or school districts want it there. In the United States, national school beverage guidelines have been successful in removing full-calorie soft drinks from schools, and replacing these with water, sports and diet drinks, and juice.[162] This is great, but of course children can still drink soft drinks outside of school, and they continue to do so in large quantities.

A survey of teenagers revealed that many teenagers find coffee repulsive, and identify coffee as a beverage that signals adulthood.[163] Fortunately for these kids, they have access to all the soda they can drink until they become adults and trade in their soda habit for a coffee habit. Children have small bodies and a lower ability to eliminate caffeine, so when they consume caffeine in moderate doses their blood levels of the drug can reach high concentrations.

It is easy for a child to get hooked on caffeine when one considers that 2-3 soft drinks a day for a child is the equivalent of 4-6 cups of coffee for an adult.[164] That is no small amount of caffeine. We all know that the consumption of soft drinks is linked to childhood obesity, and health experts have long warned that the soda industry is addicting kids to its beverages, with lifelong consequences. The conditioning that children receive from the soft drink industry may even be partly responsible for teaching them the taste and preference for sugar.

By now we've all heard about the nine teaspoons of sugar in a 12 ounce serving of soda. This added sugar, especially when it is combined with caffeine, prompts the body to produce a large amount of insulin, contributing to the insulin-induced hunger and overeating that we discussed in Chapter 4, Caffeine and Insulin. That aside, even if your insulin system works perfectly, a 12 ounce can of Coca-Cola has 140 calories, all from sugar. So even if we are to ignore all the hormonal implications of caffeine consumption, consuming caffeine from soda carries the additional consequence of shooting our bodies full of empty calories.

Before you reach for the diet soda, however, I have some bad news about that too. While the long-term general health effects of artificial sweeteners are uncertain and perhaps questionable, the effects of these sweeteners on weight loss may not be good. A one year study of 78,694 women found that those women who used artificial sweeteners were more likely to gain weight than those who did not.[165] This study concluded that the use of artificial sweeteners did not aid weight loss.

Researchers hypothesize that artificial sweeteners hinder weight loss because their sweet taste primes the body to expect incoming calories, but then when no calories are received from the apparently sweet food, the ability of the body to gauge caloric intake is lessened.[166] As our bodies get worse at measuring caloric intake by the cues we receive from our sense of taste, we become more susceptible to overeating and gain weight.

Fructose and Appetite

A large portion of the side calories we receive from caffeinated foods and beverages comes from added sugar, and this is true not only for soda, but also for just about any caffeinated beverage you can find in a supermarket refrigerator. Fructose is a constituent of this added sugar, and nutrition researchers and doctors have been giving fructose a lot of consideration recently.

The rise in obesity in recent years parallels the increasing use of fructose as a sweetener, and many health experts and researchers have begun to suspect that fructose plays a causative role in obesity. A number of studies have proven their suspicions correct. The major sources of fructose in the diet are high-fructose corn syrup, sugar, honey, fruit and fruit juice, and some vegetables. Table sugar (sucrose) is made up of roughly 50% fructose and 50% glucose. Fructose is a simple sugar like glucose, but the body reacts to fructose in a different manner.

Studies have found that fructose consumption inhibits leptin receptors, so our bodies do not get the signal that we are full and ought to reduce energy intake.[167] Instead, we keep eating. As a result, fructose, by reducing our feelings of fullness, promotes overeating. This is another explanation for the increased level of satiety that low carbohydrate dieters experience – they are eating little or no sugar, so their leptin system is working properly to suppress appetite. When high amounts of fructose (whether in high-fructose corn syrup or regular sugar form) are combined with caffeine in our favorite caffeinated beverages, the fructose and caffeine work together to destroy satiety and encourage overeating.

This helps to explain why we can drink soda after soda or sugary coffee after sugary coffee, and yet never feel full. The over consumption of sugar as a result of our caffeine addiction not only provides additional calories from sugar, but also promotes overeating generally, by decreasing our bodies' sensitivity to leptin. If you'd like to read some free, entertaining articles about fructose's assault on our waistlines written for the nutritionally-obsessed bodybuilding community, please refer to the last three sources in the following endnote.[168]

High fructose diets initiate insulin resistance in humans within short periods of time, along with rapid weight gain, high blood pressure, a preferential increase in visceral fat, and other weight-related health problems.[169] From the standpoint of overeating, the satiety-suppressive effect of fructose explains why too much of this sugar encourages overeating and contributes to both weight gain and insulin resistance.

There is growing evidence that consumption of sweetened beverages that contain fructose is associated with a high energy intake, increased body weight, and the occurrence of metabolic and cardiovascular disorders. That being said, there is not conclusive evidence that a low or moderate fructose intake has negative effects.[170] So while high amounts of fructose can contribute to overeating, weight gain, and the spot addition of central fat, you do not need to stop eating fruit!

Fruit provides a variety of beneficial nutrients, and the concentration of fructose in fruit is actually lower than its concentration in common table sugar. While you should continue to keep fruit in your diet, you should think about moderating your fruit juice intake if you drink a lot of fruit juice, as it might make the battle against overeating a losing one. A study of preschool-aged children determined that the more fruit juice children consumed, the more likely these children were to be obese and of short stature when compared to other children who consumed less juice and more milk.[171] Where you should especially avoid fructose is where it is found in foods with little to no nutritional value, such as soda and other foods that are sweetened with high-fructose corn syrup.

There is currently paranoia surrounding fructose consumption that is similar to the wholesale vilification of insulin as the cause of all weight gain. It is another effort to find the one cause of weight gain, eliminate it, and then convince readers that they can eat unlimited quantities of other foods. Fructose, however, should not be viewed outside the lens of energy balance, and its role in a weight loss diet should always be measured in its effects on overall energy intake and energy expenditure.

A reduction of dietary fructose is desirable because it will lead to a reduction in calories from the fructose itself and also to greater levels of satiety, so in these two ways the reduction of fructose reduces overeating, and brings us closer to negative energy balance. Cutting fructose intake is also important for insulin control purposes, because fructose is always packaged alongside glucose. By eliminating the sugar from our caffeinated beverages, we attack overeating by improving our insulin sensitivity, our leptin sensitivity, and by reducing the overeating of sugar calories directly by removing these calories from our diets.

Sugar Addiction

I decided to include this section because I often hear people refer to sugar as addictive, and to their difficulties in quitting sugar. Why is it so hard to quit sugar? Sugar is not biologically addictive, but many of us feel that we can't stop eating it and the foods it sweetens. If you overeat sugar in forms where it is separate from other drugs that drive your food intake such as caffeine, theobromine in chocolate, and alcohol, then this section is for you. If you are taking sugar along with a drug such as caffeine, then simply realizing that your body wants the drug more than the sugar will help you remove sugar from the equation.

If you are eating lots of sweet foods by themselves, such as cookies without chocolate, cakes without chocolate, soda without caffeine, plain vanilla ice cream, and so forth, then we need to address your issue with sugar so that we can reduce your fructose consumption and teach your body to feel full. You can try to decrease your sugar consumption over a period of time, or all at once. There are problems with doing it over time, the main one being that it is very difficult for most people to do.

While the sugar habit is not driven by biology the way other addictions are, as we eat it, we want more and more of it and food in general because it takes away our feelings of satiety via leptin resistance. So we have one bite, become more resistant to leptin, our hunger-controlling hormone, want another bite, and we get hungrier the more sugar we eat. This is why many people feel that the more they eat, the hungrier they become, and as dieters reduce their over-all food intake, they often feel their overall level of hunger decline, so long as they are not over-consuming foods high in sugar.

The best plan when dealing with sugar is to cut or even eliminate sugar in one fell swoop. Limit your daily sugar intake to one meal, or remove all of it from your kitchen at once. Throw all of it out. What works best for me is to remove all of the refined and concentrated sugar from my house, so that it's not an option for me to eat. If it's not in the house, I don't eat it.

The less sugar you eat, the less you will want sugar and food in general, because your body will regain its sensitivity to leptin and you will feel full. If you start eating sugar again, you will want more. When it comes to sugar, you will feel fuller by eating less. This works for me and everyone else that I have convinced to try a sugar reduction approach to overeating.

I never drank soda when I was growing up because my parents wouldn't let me, and I did not develop the habit of putting sugar in my hot beverages, until I became an adult. When soda and added sugars were not in my diet, I never craved them. However, when I began to consume more foods with added sugars as I got older, these foods began to occupy a larger and larger space in my diet over time. Let sugar know that it's unwelcome in your kitchen, de-sugar your life, and experience the results. Furthermore, if you take most of the sugar out of your diet you'll see there is not much left for you to overeat anyway. Just about everything that's left is good for you, and relatively low in calories.

When Getting Fat is Healthy

Why is fructose such a nightmare if it's available in fruit? Shouldn't we have adapted to it by now? Why isn't it good for us? Well it is. Or rather, it was, sometimes. Confused? Don't worry; our discussion will get interesting in a minute. As we have already discussed, there are times when having extra body fat is beneficial for survival. Moderate levels of body fat are a significant biological advantage for surviving the winter, a time when, before modernization, food was scarce.

The fittest among our ancestors may have evolved an ability to store fat before winter, based on environmental cues which signaled the changing of the seasons. The cues included diminishing sunlight and perhaps an abundance of sweet fruit in the late summer and fall in seasonal climates. When our ancestors' bodies took in these cues, it was a signal for their bodies to shift into winter metabolism, and increase hunger so that we could overeat and put on fat for the winter.

To this day, our bodies continue to shift into overeating mode when given the environmental cues of high fructose consumption and declining levels of sunlight. The large amounts of fructose we currently consume might be telling our prehistoric bodies that winter is coming and that we should overeat as much as we can while food is available.

Of course, our bodies don't know that the world has changed so much that the fructose it is getting is now available year-round in huge quantities and no longer signals a coming winter. For those of us who live in the industrialized world, this winter metabolism is obsolete. The winter metabolism theory still awaits confirmation, but until then, it remains an interesting theory that adds perspective to our dietary woes.

A Little Heartburn

There is one more way in which caffeine causes side calories to creep into your diet, and it is devious. Caffeine and caffeine-containing beverages cause the overproduction of

105

stomach acid in some people, and it is this phenomenon that is responsible for the heartburn and acid indigestion that can accompany caffeine intake. In order to deal with this problem, many people eat something with their coffee or tea in an effort to settle their stomachs – usually a bagel, donut, or other pastry –further increasing their energy intakes.

Summary

Caffeine is an addictive drug that programs us, mostly through negative reinforcement, to acquire a taste for the foods and beverages that carry it. When we consume caffeinated foods and beverages for our regular fix, we expose ourselves to all of the side calories that come with caffeine, usually in the form of fat and sugar. These side calories significantly increase our daily energy intakes, contributing to positive energy balance and creating weight gain over time.

The fructose that is part of the sugar side calories presents additional problems for the dieter, because fructose disrupts our feeling of satiety, promoting overeating. Removing sugar from your caffeinated foods and beverages is a good step toward weight loss, and this strategy will be explored in more detail in Chapter 8, Optimal Caffeine Use. In the next chapter, we will finish our discussion of the negative implications of caffeine consumption for the energy balance of a dieter who is trying to lose weight.

CHAPTER 6
DIET PILLS, GREEN TEA, AND THE THYROID

Advertising is the art of making whole lies out of half truths.

-Edgar A. Shoaff

In this chapter we will take one final look at how some caffeinated beverages can contribute to positive energy balance and weight gain by decreasing the body's resting metabolic rate in those individuals who are sensitive to this effect. As we noted in the first chapter, most of the blame that our resting metabolic rates receive for causing weight gain has no foundation. The overwhelming majority of overweight and obese individuals have faster resting metabolic rates than lean individuals, due to the increased fat-free mass that heavier individuals carry.

And yet we turn to pills and elixirs that promise to increase our resting metabolic rates to youthful levels, when most of us have normal metabolisms. So why this chapter? In part it is to address the elephant in the room that is the diet pill industry, which claims that caffeine burns fat, and in part to speak to the rare dieter who actually does have a slow metabolism (or who strongly insists that he does), and seeks to attend to this problem.

The media constantly bombards us with the notion that caffeine burns fat and boosts metabolism, and that we should increase our consumption of at least one source of caffeine, green tea. The fitness and health industries revere green tea as a magical elixir or health, vitality, weight loss, and any other desirable attributes they can think of. The reverence green tea receives is reminiscent of the following statement made by Dr. Cornelius Buntekuh in the seventeenth century:

> We advise tea for the whole nation and for every nation. We advise men and women to drink tea daily; hour by hour if possible; beginning with ten cups a day, and increasing the dose to the utmost quantity that the stomach can contain and the kidneys eliminate.

Please note that Dr. Buntekuh (who reportedly drank up to 200 cups of tea per day himself) was paid by the Dutch East India Company, so he was a physician compensated by a company that not coincidentally was trying to sell as much tea as possible.[172] Due in part to his overzealous tea consumption, Buntekuh died early at the age of 38. Although he did not die of illness – he fell down a staircase while carrying books – it is fair to speculate that his frazzled nerves, jitters, and sleep deprivation contributed to his unsteady footing.[173]

Today, the caffeine industries continue to compensate medical professionals and spend millions of dollars funding studies to produce research favorable to caffeine and the foods and beverages that carry this drug.[174] This is not something I want to spend much time on except in instances where it is highly entertaining (as with Dr. Buntekuh) being that the sources I cite give the issue of research funding for favorable research outcomes a thorough treatment.

Whole Lies Out of Half-Truths

Despite all of the fattening effects of caffeine that we have discussed up to this point, does caffeine in green tea form actually warrant the worship it receives today? Why is caffeine a part of most weight loss supplements? Well, a number of studies bear out the metabolism-boosting effects of large amounts of caffeine, these effects being dependent on the amount of caffeine consumed.[175]

When we drink several cups of coffee, we can expect a small boost in metabolic rate for the next few hours. For this reason, health experts sometimes recommend caffeine as an addition to a weight loss diet, and this is where the "caffeine for weight loss" industry makes whole lies out of half-truths. How much caffeine do you need to consume to get a metabolic boost, and how big is that metabolic boost? And what part of the data are diet pill manufacturers obscuring?

Before we begin answering these questions, let's touch base once more with the finding that increasing the body's resting metabolic rate is not the best way to devise a weight loss plan. All of the research that we have discussed points to decreasing energy intake, increasing energy expenditure through exercise, but not increasing resting energy expenditure (metabolism), because resting energy expenditure contributes less than food intake and exercise in affecting overall energy balance. Slow metabolism is not the reason for weight gain in the first place, and very few of us actually need to speed up our metabolisms. But enough of that, let's address the above questions.

First, to get a meaningful metabolic boost from caffeine, you will have to consume 4 mg per pound of your body weight. So if you weigh 150 pounds, that comes out to 600 mg of caffeine, or six cups of coffee. If you weigh 200 pounds, then you will have to consume 800 mg of caffeine, or 8 cups of coffee. That is a lot of caffeine. That is an amount of caffeine that most people can not comfortably consume in one sitting on a regular basis.

If you can take that dose, however, you can expect about a 13% boost in your resting metabolic rate for a period of time, at best until the end of the day following your drinking of 6-8 cups of coffee. Your body will burn fat at a faster rate, picking up fat from its stores and re-depositing most of it (probably in your midsection) but successfully burning up some of it. It's not perfect, but it sounds alright so far: we will get some fat-burning out of the whole deal if we can tolerate the large dose of caffeine required, but there is more.

Second, and more importantly, the researchers who study caffeine's metabolic effects are careful to point out an important consideration. Caffeine's efficacy as a metabolism booster is dependent on an absence of a compensatory increase in food intake that takes place with the increase in caffeine intake.[176] In other words, large amounts of caffeine may help boost your metabolism some, but this effect can be blunted or eliminated entirely by a simultaneous increase in your food intake, if caffeine increases your appetite.

If caffeine intake brings with it an increased food intake, any positive metabolic effects are lost. The problem with the studies that find a metabolic boost from caffeine consumption is that they are narrow in time, and examine the body's rate of fat-burning in the *hours* after caffeine consumption, and do not examine any changes in eating patterns that occur after the high caffeine dose that is needed to increase fat-burning.

For some hours after a large dose of caffeine, the body burns fat faster than it usually does, and that's where the studies stop. They neither look at changes in food intake that accompany the large dose of caffeine, nor do they look at changes in food intake that follow the period of increased fat-burning. The researchers do acknowledge that more study is necessary in this area, and that a key assumption of caffeine's efficacy as a fat-burner is the lack of an accompanying hunger-stimulating effect. But, as we have seen, caffeine ingestion causes increases in appetite through multiple biological pathways, breaks down muscle (leading to long-term metabolic slowdown), and brings with it a large amount of side calories, so it is unlikely that any beneficial metabolic benefits from imbibing large quantities of the drug survive. That is what the "caffeine for weight loss" sellers understandably don't want you to know.

Weight Loss Supplements and Appetite

Taking caffeine for weight loss is impractical from the standpoint of increasing resting energy expenditure, but what about taking caffeine for appetite suppression? Most of the weight loss supplements on the market contain caffeine, usually with the addition of another stimulant for synergistic effect, and these supplements promise to blunt your appetite. This sounds promising because less appetite means lower energy intake, and that is arguably the best way to lose weight and maintain leanness. Let's refocus on the chronically elevated cortisol levels that result from regular caffeine use, which impede weight loss while encouraging weight gain.

It is true that some people find stimulants useful for appetite suppression, but the way stimulants suppress appetite

111

is by putting the body into panic mode and simply delaying eating until later, when hunger comes back even stronger to compensate for the body's perceived stress. While some people on diet pills may find appetite suppression help-ful, in the long-term these stimulant pills are harming the body's ability to stay at a healthy weight by, among other things, increasing our levels of cortisol, which promote overeating and muscle wasting.

The problem with stimulant pills for weight loss is that even though there is some evidence of a short-term benefit for weight loss, there is no evidence of a long-term benefit. On the contrary, there is mounting evidence that stimulants bring about bouts of binge eating, which could negate all of the benefits of using stimulants for weight loss.[177]

While caffeine and other stimulants are associated with binge eating and fatty food cravings in studies, it is likely that this phenomenon varies among individuals, so you can be the best judge of what happens to your appetite when you vary your caffeine intake. You may find that you barely want to eat at all once you cut caffeine, as is the case for me.

In the 1990s, herbal weight loss pills containing a combi-nation of caffeine and ephedrine became popular. A study was done on this stimulant combination to determine how helpful it would be for preventing the weight gain experi-enced by individuals who quit smoking.[178] Smoking ces-sation is usually associated with weight gain, and the 225 volunteers in the study were heavy smokers who wanted to quit without gaining weight in the process.

The weight gain in the group treated with the stimulant combination was less than the weight gain in the untreated group during the first 12 weeks of the study. Sounds like good news for the stimulant pushers, but not so fast. A one year follow-up revealed that both groups had experienced the same amount of weight gain by the end of that year.

In other words, the caffeine and ephedrine combination worked in the short-term to suppress appetite, but this stimulant combination did nothing to stave off weight gain in the long-term. The stimulant treated group caught up to the weight gain of the untreated group so that both groups ended up with similar weight gains at the end of the year.

The ephedrine-caffeine combination is often used by body-builders as a fat-burning aid, with aspirin added in as well. This supposed fat burning bundle is known as an ECA (Ephedrine, Caffeine, Aspirin) stack. It is no wonder that these fat-burning pills are popular, as everyone is looking for a quick fix. A cursory internet search reveals page after page claiming that caffeine and ephedrine, when combined, make for the "ideal diet pill." As we have seen, however, the beneficial short-term effects of stimulant pills for weight loss do not hold up in the long-term, and now that we have gone over the roles that cortisol plays in weight gain, it is easy to understand why.

Diet pills are too good to be true - not to mention all the un-fortunate individuals who were duped into buying diet pills (often based on an ECA stack with added stimulants) that ended up dying from liver failure or needing a liver trans-plant to survive. It is ironic, given the weight gain-promot-ing qualities of caffeine we've discussed in the previous chapters, that it is often advertised as a magical fat-burn ing pill and found in a large number of fat-burning supple-ments. Stimulant diet pills are not the way to achieve more favorable levels of energy balance for weight loss.

As for green tea in particular, researchers have found that the metabolism-boosting effects of green tea cannot be explained by its caffeine content alone.[179] In human trials, treatment with 50 mg caffeine alone (the amount equivalent to that found in the green tea extract used in this study) had no effect on energy expenditure, whereas treatment with the green tea extract resulted in increased energy expenditure.[180] It should be no surprise that 50 mg of caffeine, the amount found in half a cup of coffee, had no effect on energy expenditure, given our above discussion of the huge amounts of caffeine we must ingest to experience a metabolic boost.

This finding suggests that the plant compounds in green tea are the active ingredients that have beneficial effects for weight loss. Specifically, it is the tea catechins that researchers believe are responsible for green tea's metabolism-boosting effects.[181] The finding that plant substances can be beneficial for weight loss should be no surprise, but what is surprising in this study is that a small amount of caffeine had no effect in speeding metabolism; all of the weight loss benefits came from the tea's catechin content. Animal studies support a role for catechins in promoting weight loss, and apart from tea, catechins can be found in fruits and berries.[182]

The Nail in the Supplement Coffin

In two very recent studies, the most extensive studies of the effectiveness of weight loss supplements to date, researchers found no significant weight loss benefit from any weight loss supplements, caffeinated or not.[183] The studies evaluated polyglucosamide, cabbage powder, konjak extract, sodiumalginate-complex, bean concentrate, L-carnitine, fiber formulation, guarana seed powder (a concentrated source of caffeine), selected plant extracts, guar gum, chromium picolinate, ephedra, ephedrine, bitter orange, conjugated linoleic acid (CLA), calcium, glucomannan, chitosan, and green tea.

114

Guess what? The only thing these supplements are good at shrinking is your wallet. The amount of money Europeans and Americans spend on weight loss supplements each year is about three billion dollars combined, and it turns out that these supplements have no effect. These newer studies looked at actual weight loss at the end of the study, rather than at the change in fat-burning right after a supplement such as caffeine is consumed. Even if caffeine does increase your rate of fat-burning after you take it, this does not help you lose weight if your energy balance remains even or positive. Be wary of supplements.

Fluoride and the Thyroid

Let's return to green tea and look at it from a different angle now. Even if green tea does have some minor health benefits, for the rare metabolically-challenged dieter, the dangers of green tea may outweigh these benefits. If you suspect or know that your metabolism is slow, I recommend avoiding green and black teas as much as possible, and having these beverages only in small amounts and irregularly.

I hesitate to make this recommendation because I have always liked the taste of black tea compared to coffee, and my cultural heritage prizes tea, so to some degree I feel uncomfortable speaking out against this dietary mainstay. That being said, teas are inferior to chocolate and coffee as caffeine sources because of the high levels of fluoride that accumulate in tea leaves. Fluoride can have significant negative effects on your thyroid, a gland that plays a critical role in regulating metabolism.

The thyroid gland is an endocrine gland in your neck that makes two thyroid hormones. About 93% of the hormones the thyroid makes is T4 (thyroxine, the inactive form), and 7% is T3 (the active form). The T4 is made in the thyroid and the liver converts T4 to T3. The main role of these thyroid hormones is to regulate metabolism by controlling the rate at which your cells use energy. If your thyroid hormones are not at healthy levels, your body's cells will not be burning energy at an optimal rate.

The classic symptoms of an underactive thyroid, known as hypothyroidism, are weight gain, fatigue, feeling cold, swelling, dry skin, soft nails, hair loss, constipation, muscle cramps, impaired memory, and depression. Some hypothyroid patients have trouble losing weight, even with low calorie diets and exercise. Hypothyroidism reduces energy expenditure, so the thyroid is important to think about if you are metabolically challenged.

Risk factors for developing hypothyroidism include: having a family member with a history of thyroid problems, smoking, past treatment with lithium or amiodarone, living in an area where the soil is low in iodine (the "Goiter Belt" in the Midwestern United States), heavy soy consumption, exposure to fluoride, being female, autoimmune disease (especially Hashimoto's), past treatment with radioactive iodine, and congenital hypothyroidism (being born hypothyroid).

Some nutritionists suspect that a large number of people with an underactive thyroid are not diagnosed. The main reason for this is that doctors don't agree on the best way to diagnose and treat people with sub-clinical hypothyroidism, a subtle underactive thyroid. While it is easier to recognize a person with full-blown hypothyroidism, subtle hypothyroidism is harder to recognize, and symptoms such as weight gain and fatigue can be attributed to a large number of other causes. Let's get to what all of this has to do with tea, the most popular beverage in the world after water.

The tea leaves used to make the green and black tea that we drink contain large amounts of fluoride, because tea accumulates more fluoride than any other edible plant.[184] Fluoride can alter thyroid function, and depending on exposure levels can lead to hypothyroidism. In the past, before the dangers of the practice were revealed, European doctors used fluoride as a treatment for hyperthyroidism, an overactive thyroid. Fluoride was used because it was found to be effective at reducing thyroid activity.

Not only does fluoride intake inhibit conversion of T4 to T3, but it also decreases levels of both T4 and T3.[185] Estimates of the fluoride content of tea leaves vary, but the research suggests that if you are a heavy tea drinker, your fluoride intake may reach toxic levels.[186] Ironically, health experts recommend heavy consumption of tea, especially green tea, as a panacea. In response to these recommendations, some critics of "healthful" tea consumption refer to this practice as a "health fad from hell."

A study of tea drinking in children found that the average fluoride levels in tea were 2.36 mg/L, and that regular tea intake put these children at risk for fluoride's toxic effects.[187] This level of fluoride is still within the EPA's maximum contaminant level of 4 mg/L, but it is above the EPA's secondary maximum contaminant level of 2 mg/L, which is a non-enforceable guideline aimed at limiting the undesirable effects of fluoride exposure such as skin and tooth discoloration.

The fluoride level of tea varies widely, however, and can sometimes be as high as 9 mg/L.[188] If you do a cursory internet search on fluoride levels in tea, you will find that the fluoride level of 2.36 mg/L that I use as a baseline reference here is on the low side. But even the low estimates are high enough to cause significant metabolic effects, especially if

117

you subscribe to the green and black tea health claims, and consume large amounts of tea.

Tea producers and marketers have long advertised the fluoride content of their teas as beneficial, so it's not as if they ever denied the presence of fluoride in tea. In response, consumer advocates questioned the healthfulness of green tea and its high fluoride content. I recommend that you read *Green Tea, Fluoride & the Thyroid,* which is available online, if you are interested in learning more about fluoride's dark side, and our exposure to fluoride in tea.[189] The author cites extensive research on fluoride's negative health effects and the high level of fluoride exposure that tea consumption presents.

In 2006, the National Research Council (NRC), arguably the highest scientific authority of the United States, published a report entitled, *Fluoride in Drinking Water: A Scientific Review of EPA's Standards.* In the report, NRC researchers connected fluoride with a number of health problems, and in many ways the report is a wake-up call on the issue of fluoride safety. For our purposes, we will focus on the researchers' findings on fluoride's effects on the thyroid.

The NRC found that fluoride has effects on the thyroid at varying levels of intake (both high and low), and that chronic exposure to fluoride altered thyroid hormone levels to those seen in early and full hypothyroidism.[190] The researchers noted the anti-hyperthyroid effects of fluoride as well as the mineral's inhibiting effect on the conversion of T4 to T3 to explain its negative effects. The NRC also noted that the recent decline in U.S. iodine intake can increase fluoride's thyroid-damaging effects.[191]

Cortisol Strikes Again

Unfortunately, it is time to revisit cortisol, now in relation to the thyroid gland. In addition to all of the previously described negative effects of a chronically elevated cortisol level, we can now add the inhibition of thyroid stimulating hormone (TSH).[192] A high stress level, as we have long suspected, really is bad for everything. TSH is the primary regulator of thyroid function, signaling the body to produce T4 and T3. In a healthy individual, low levels of T4 and T3 signal the production of TSH, which in turn signals the production of T4 and T3.

If high cortisol levels prevent the production of TSH, your thyroid will not be producing enough T4 and T3. Furthermore, excessive cortisol levels (just as fluoride intake) may also suppress the action of the enzyme that converts T4 to T3, the active form.[193] The result of all of this is that your thyroid is under-producing the hormones with which it regulates your body's metabolism. The effects of fluoride on your thyroid are more than enough by themselves to keep your metabolism sluggish, but if you are a heavy tea drinker you are not only getting thyroidal detriments from fluoride, but also from the caffeine-induced high cortisol levels.

Some nutritionists also believe that by putting stress on your liver, caffeine directly impairs the efficient conversion of T4 to T3, or impairs the release of T3 from the liver, contributing to non-optimal thyroid hormone levels and a lower resting metabolic rate than would exist if the liver were not busy detoxifying and eliminating caffeine. There is some research to support reasoning in this direction, but none involving caffeine. The levels of T3 being made in or released from the liver are reduced by liver damage and impairment, such as that which is present in alcoholism and chemical exposure.[194]

However, there is no research evidence that caffeine, even in large amounts, damages or impairs the liver, except where it is taken in conjunction with painkillers such as acetaminophen. It is not clear to what degree caffeine is a burden on the liver, and to what degree the liver's detoxification and elimination of caffeine impairs the liver's maintenance of healthy thyroid hormone levels. Caffeine can have negative effects on thyroid hormone levels when it is taken in the form of tea and through its stimulation of cortisol release, but it is still uncertain if there are negative effects that arise directly from caffeine's detoxification and elimination by the liver.

Improving Thyroid Function

If you know or suspect that your thyroid function is weak, there are some steps you can take to strengthen this gland. If you have known problems with your thyroid, please consult with your doctor before implementing any of the following recommendations.

First, normal thyroid function requires sufficient iodine intake. Make sure that there are a few iodine sources that are a regular part of your diet. Notable sources include iodized salt, seaweed, fish and seafood, and dairy products. As for fish and seafood, if you choose to consume foods from this category on a regular basis, try to avoid larger fish and favor smaller fish such as sardines, wild salmon, herring, anchovies, tilapia, and cod. Unfortunately, due to mercury contamination, larger fish should not be consumed regularly.

Please be aware that the decision to eat fish and seafood may require some more careful consideration in the near future, as our oceans become more polluted over time. Mercury is not the only seafood contaminant we need to worry about, but this is not a book about seafood. For more information about safe fish and seafood consumption, seafood contaminants and the contamination of the oceans in general, please see the references in the following endnote.[195]

Second, avoid unnecessary sources of fluoride, such as tea. You don't need to give up this beverage forever, but make sure that you are drinking it in moderation, and not in accordance with Dr. Buntekuh's recommendations. Instead of drinking lots of tea, choose foods with high levels of antioxidants to receive the same benefits of tea consumption without the fluoride. Herbal teas, fruits, berries, greens, and vegetables can provide all of the antioxidants you need to live a healthy life.

Third, try to make exercise a regular part of your routine. Exercise stimulates the thyroid gland's secretion of hormones and increases the sensitivity of the body's cells to the effects of the thyroid gland. And of course, exercise itself burns calories, adding to your energy expenditure further.

Fluoride and Testosterone

Healthy testosterone levels are important for supporting a healthy sex drive in both men and women, and for maintaining muscle mass. The maintenance of muscle mass throughout life is of vital importance for maintaining a desirable level of resting energy expenditure. The bodybuilding community has long been suspicious of green tea's effects on testosterone levels, and with good cause.

Healthy testosterone levels are of central importance for people who are trying to build and maintain high levels of muscle mass. The plant substances in green tea (polyphenols in this instance), which give green tea some of its benefits, also lower testosterone production.[196] The suppression of testosterone production is dose dependent, so

121

the more green tea you drink, the lower your testosterone levels will become.

As if that was not enough, fluoride also lowers testosterone levels![197] In addition and in part due to its testosterone-lowering effects, a high fluoride intake is also associated with infertility and other reproductive problems. So not only does caffeine lower testosterone levels by stimulating cortisol production, it also does so through fluoride intake when taken in the form of green or black tea. The lower our levels of muscle-building testosterone, the lower our overall muscle mass will be, and the more difficult it will be to maintain a lean weight at similar levels of energy intake. Alright, I'm tired of bearing all this bad news. Let's talk about an interesting new theory instead.

Deficiency-Driven Overeating

There is a theory floating around the medical and nutrition communities which states that at least some overeating is the result of nutrient deficiencies. The theory is that we overeat in part because our bodies are looking for certain nutrients that we require for health. There is a related nutritional observation that lends some support to this theory. Weight loss researchers have observed that we tend to eat more when we are presented with a variety of foods to choose from, and the more variety they give us, the more we eat.

Many of us recognize this fact of eating as the "buffet phenomenon." When we're at a buffet and have many foods to choose from, we must try many, if not all of them, regardless of whether we are hungry or not - not to mention dessert, which goes into a different stomach altogether.

Some researchers believe this is the case because we are evolutionarily wired to seek out food variety in order to get all the nutrients we need and increase our chances of survival. The researchers performed an experiment where they set out two bowls of chocolate candy for passersby to eat. In one bowl the candies were all one color, and in the other bowl the candies were multi-colored. The result was that the multi-colored candies were consumed twice as fast. When there is variety, the researchers found, we eat 30% more than when there is not.[198]

Other research has shown that when we expose ourselves to several different flavors at the same time, our brains tell us to keep eating.[199] While this does not prove that we over-eat in an effort to correct nutritional deficiencies, it does suggest some evolutionary motives behind our eating be-havior which go beyond just filling up on calories. If this mechanism exists, it once helped us to eat a variety of fruits and vegetables, and had healthful consequences. Now, this same mechanism may inspire us to overeat a variety of junk foods (of which there is now a very large variety), resulting in weight gain and its associated health problems.

Does caffeine contribute to nutritional deficiencies which might lead us to overeat in seeking out those nutrients? As it turns out, caffeinated beverages do inhibit the absorp-tion of some nutrients, most notably iron. Perhaps if we become iron deficient, our bodies go into overeating mode in order to try to compensate for the deficiency. Perhaps not. As to an underactive thyroid and overeating, some individuals with underactive thyroids find that they can't help but binge eat.

Perhaps our bodies, sensing that we need more iodine and other thyroid supportive nutrients to get our metabolism back in gear, spur us to overeat. I am not aware of any con-clusive research on deficiency-driven overeating, so for now this will have to remain food for thought. You can overeat that all you want.

Since we just discussed the theory of deficiency-driven overeating, I think it is appropriate to mention here that some nutritionists believe some overeating is the result of dehydration. The theory goes that we are thirsty, and rather than drink to relieve our thirst, we eat to relieve our thirst instead. While I am not sure to what extent we mistake thirst for hunger, I think this theory holds some water because as a diuretic, caffeine does contribute to dehydration, and if we choose to relieve this dehydration by drinking large quantities of sugary beverages rather than water, then caffeine can contribute to "dehydration-driven overeating."

This is something to consider if you are a regular caffeine consumer and find that you are often very thirsty, and proceed to quench your thirst with calorie-filled drinks rather than with water. The corrective measure here, other than the elimination of the cause of this dehydration, is to prefer water over other beverages as your thirst quencher.

Summary

For the dieter who seeks to increase his resting energy expenditure, caffeinated weight loss supplements do not offer an effective strategy. First, the use of caffeine for weight loss requires a very large intake of caffeine for a modest increase in energy expenditure. Second, the use of caffeine for weight loss does not take into account the compensatory overeating and muscle breakdown that caffeine consumption stimulates. Furthermore, resting energy expenditure augmentation is not the proper focus for weight loss, whereas energy intake and energy expenditure in exercise are.

That aside, for the dieter who is concerned about his resting energy expenditure, a moderate or high intake of tea may be detrimental, due to the high total fluoride intake that liberal consumption of tea provides. Fluoride negatively affects thyroid function, and the thyroid is instrumental in regulating resting energy expenditure. A healthy thyroid requires adequate amounts of iodine, exercise, and an absence of high levels of fluoride in the diet.

A high intake of green tea and a high fluoride intake also lower testosterone levels, making it more difficult to maintain the muscle mass which is responsible for most of your resting energy expenditure. The takeaway point here is to practice moderation with tea consumption, to be wary of products that promise an easy fix, and to be wary of the promotion of the extreme consumption of any food or beverage.

This chapter ends our examination of caffeine's effects on energy intake and energy expenditure. Now we will move on to how we can apply all of this information in order to get leaner and stay that way.

CHAPTER 7
THE DECAF PLAN

All over the world, people drink it, blindly, by the millions, by the hundreds of millions, by the billions. *And they must have it, they think they cannot do without it.*
-Mark Helprin, *Memoir from Antproof Case* (1995)

This book is called *The Decaf Diet* because its main strategy is that of promoting weight loss by slowly decaffeinating your body, thereby removing the problems of overeating and a slowed resting metabolic rate that caffeine creates. By removing some or all of the caffeine from your diet and decaffeinating your life, you will come closer to the type of health that the human organism enjoyed before the advent of caffeine use.

From an evolutionary perspective, which you already know I believe is a helpful lens in thinking about diet and nutrition, caffeine entered the human diet very recently. It is reasonable to assume, therefore, that we are not as well adapted to it as we are to water, which we have been imbibing since our earliest origins. I believe that the more closely we can approximate our original diets and lifestyle habits (without going to extremes), the better quality of life we will be able to enjoy.

That being said, quitting caffeine can be a very difficult process, depending on how you do it. Going cold turkey by switching straight to water can be an excruciatingly painful experience for some people. For others, weaning themselves off of caffeine gradually is an impossibility, due to their vulnerability to the drug's reinforcing effects, and they find going cold turkey to be the preferable quitting method. Some people experience rather severe withdrawal symptoms when they try to stop consuming caffeine, and others feel little or nothing. If you choose to reduce your caffeine consumption based on the information in the previous chapters, you can choose between a gradual reduction of caffeine, quitting cold turkey, and in-between variants.

There are a few things you should know before you begin on either path. First, unlike quitting caffeine cold turkey, a gradual reduction in caffeine consumption is not associated with *any* withdrawal symptoms.[200] So you can reduce and completely eliminate your consumption of caffeine over a period of weeks or months with virtually no unpleasant withdrawal symptoms. But consider again, that is only if you can actually carry out a gradual reduction.

If you find that you are the type of caffeine consumer such that when you have one cup of coffee, you must have another, and then another, and another, this strategy will not work for you. I find that the reinforcing effects of caffeine affect me strongly, such that my cravings for caffeine increase with each dose of the drug, and it is easier for me to quit by avoiding it altogether. But not everyone feels that way, so I will describe both strategies and you can pick the one that works best for you.

If you don't want any part in a caffeine reduction strategy, the next chapter will describe how to continue to consume caffeine while reducing its negative effects for your appetite, resting energy expenditure, and the relocation of fat stores. I recommend that you still read through this chapter for general information on alternative beverages and dietary and lifestyle aids that you can implement whether or not you decide to reduce your current caffeine consumption. Specifically, the Mood Support and Exercise sections are equally applicable to the following chapter, and rather than reproduce the same sections in two chapters, I will refer back to this chapter for these lifestyle aid sections if you skip it. Furthermore, you may find some of the beverage suggestions below interesting, even if you don't reduce your caffeine intake.

Some nutritionists maintain that the effects of caffeine are cumulative, and that it may take heavy coffee drinkers up to a week to fully eliminate the drug from their bodies.[201] That's if you go cold turkey, however, so with a gradual reduction it will take longer. The fact that most of us have another dose of caffeine before our bodies have completely eliminated the previous dose lends support to this theory of caffeine accumulation in the body's tissues. This suggests that coming off of caffeine will take longer depending on how long you have been using it, and also that the effects of caffeine consumption add up over time.

As you do reduce your caffeine consumption, you will experience an overall decrease in your cortisol levels, and a corresponding decrease in your feelings of stress. Over time, your stress threshold will improve, and events that stress you out when you are caffeinated will not have the same effect on you when you reduce or eliminate your caffeine consumption. You will also be less prone to stress-induced and insulin-induced overeating and will be better able to maintain your fat-burning muscle mass.

If you have problems with insulin resistance or low blood sugar and rebound overeating, cutting your caffeine intake can help tremendously, as it did for me. Cutting your caffeine intake will also reduce your exposure to side calories, especially fructose, which has the dual effect of increasing your energy intake directly and decreasing your feelings of satiety through leptin resistance. Just by virtue of reducing your caffeine intake, you can significantly decrease your energy intake while increasing your energy expenditure. With that enticement, let's talk about how to best reduce our caffeine intakes.

Gradual Reduction

There are a number of ways to go about gradually reducing the caffeine in your diet. You can simply reduce your caffeine intake by a certain amount per day or per week, until you have reduced your consumption enough to experience weight loss. Or, you can do a similar reduction and also replace one of your former cups of coffee with a caffeine-free beverage.

This is the easier strategy because it allows you to keep part of your caffeine ritual intact, that of drinking a hot or cold beverage at specific points in the day. If you get your caffeine from a variety of sources, you can cut out the most concentrated sources first. Start by eliminating coffee, then eliminate black tea, and so forth. If you are a tea drinker you can start by brewing your tea for shorter amounts of time, switch to green, then to white, and then cut it off altogether.

For example, if you drink four cups of coffee per day, you can begin your gradual reduction by cutting back to three or three and a half cups per day, and replace the missing coffee with some decaf or a different beverage. After you get used to drinking three cups of coffee per day, you can decrease your consumption further, to two cups per day. At that point you'll be drinking two cups of coffee and two cups of a replacement beverage, and so forth.

In the alternative, you can start with your four cups of coffee and progressively weaken them by mixing in decaf, until you are drinking all decaf in your coffee mug. The length of time that it takes to comfortably make this reduction will vary among individuals. The best part is that as long as you can stick to this or a similar gradual reduction strategy, you will wean yourself off of caffeine without the usual withdrawal symptoms.

Replacing some of your caffeinated beverages with caffeine-free beverages has the added benefit of providing antioxidants and other beneficial plant compounds that are present in coffee and tea, so that you don't lose the beneficial aspects of your previous caffeine consumption. For those of us who partake in a daily caffeine ritual, conserving parts of that ritual helps to make for a comfortable reduction of caffeine intake. After the turkey note that follows, I'll describe a number of tasty and nutritious caffeine-free beverages that you can add into your schedule in place of one (and eventually all) of your caffeinated drinks.

Turkeys and Semi-Turkeys

Now let's talk about how to quit cold turkey or make a sudden downshift in your caffeine consumption. If you find it easier, as I do, to quit all at once, rather than gradually, there are a few points to consider. The advantage in quitting all at once is that you are on the road to caffeine-free weight loss much faster, but you have to put up with the full onslaught of withdrawal symptoms. I've done it numerous times myself both in doing my research for this book and before I ever contemplated coming up with a caffeine reduction plan.

Going cold turkey can get harder both with age and with increasing quantities of caffeine consumption, but for those of us who can't quit caffeine gradually, I'll describe how you can get through a cold turkey caffeine elimination while minimizing or even avoiding the pain of withdrawal.

If you go from ten cups of coffee a day to zero overnight, you will probably die. Well ok you won't die, but you'll want to. If you are dropping from one or two cups of coffee a day to zero overnight, this is much more manageable, but you might still suffer a little. Fatigue is usually the first withdrawal symptom, followed by headache. Withdrawal symptoms usually appear 12-24 hours after caffeine discontinuation and peak 8-16 hours later; headaches disappear after a few days and other symptoms weaken over time.[202]

To minimize the withdrawal symptoms that you experience, you're going to need nutritional support and rest. Ideally, if you have the time, you can sleep through your withdrawal symptoms. Most of us don't have the time to sleep for several days, however, and some of us will experience strong headaches and insomnia rather than fatigue when we quit, so sleeping through it is not an option for everyone.

Exercise and liberal water drinking can help accelerate the detoxification process and may help you recover your natural energy levels more quickly. However, be warned that exercise, especially strenuous exercise, can make some of your withdrawal symptoms worse. Exercise can make your headache worse, because it will increase circulation throughout your body and your brain is already experiencing more blood flow than it is used to, now that you've cut caffeine. So be careful with exercising too much while going cold turkey. Other than that, focus on fresh fruits and vegetables, water, the beverages described below, and rest. You will get through it.

There's also an interesting exercise twist that can be helpful for quitting cold turkey. If you are a regular exerciser, you are already counteracting the blood vessel-constricting and circulation-reducing effects of caffeine consumption. As a result, your circulation while you consume caffeine may be similar to your circulation off of caffeine, so if you quit cold turkey, you might not even get the infamous headache!

This is why those of us who exercise regularly find it easier to quit caffeine, because the withdrawal symptoms are not as strong and therefore do not have as much power to pull us back into the habit. Now that we have gone over the two methods that you can use to reduce your caffeine intake, let's discuss some replacement beverages.

Decaf Brews

Decaffeinated coffee, tea, and caffeine-free sodas are good first steps to take on the way to decaffeinating your diet. Keep in mind, however, that decaffeinated coffee and tea are not caffeine-free. There is still some residual caffeine left in decaffeinated products, but it is much less than in the fully caffeinated versions. The decaffeinated and caffeine-free versions of your favorite caffeinated beverages can be an important aid in your effort to stop using caffeine because you get a similar (but reduced) taste experience and can keep much of your existing caffeine ritual intact.

That being said, you already know that in general, I do not recommend green or black tea in large amounts, whether decaffeinated or regular, due to its fluoride content. I also do not recommend sugary sodas, due to their high fructose content. However, for a short period of time while you are decreasing your caffeine intake, these decaffeinated replacement beverages can be helpful as temporary, transitional tools.

The typical methods of decaffeination involve the use of a chemical solvent to remove caffeine from coffee beans or tea leaves. After the solvent has done its work, it is rinsed off. Small amounts of solvent remain, however, and this has caused concern among decaffeinated coffee and tea drinkers for some time. The most common solvent used for decaffeination is methylene chloride.[203]

Most decaffeinated coffee and tea contain some residual methylene chloride, and methylene chloride is carcinogenic. Whether the amounts that are left in decaffeinated products are safe for consumption is the subject of some debate, but if you want to be on the safe side, you should consume decaffeinated beverages in moderation, or find a brand that is free from chemical residues.

There are some solvent-free methods of decaffeination that use water or carbon dioxide to remove caffeine. Finding out which brands are decaffeinated without solvents requires a little bit of research, but if you consume a lot of decaffeinated coffee or tea and are concerned about lingering chemical residues, then you might want to look into the brand you are currently drinking.

Unfortunately and predictably, most of the major decaffeinated brands are chemically decaffeinated. Your best bet for chemical-free decaffeinated coffee will be a brand that uses the Swiss Water Process or CO_2 (carbon dioxide) extraction for decaffeination. In New York, I often encounter Swiss Water Process decaffeinated coffee in coffeehouses, so this type of decaf is not completely obscure.

If you are a tea drinker, I am not aware of any solvent-free decaffeinated teas on the market, but they may exist. The Swiss Water Process and carbon dioxide extraction methods are viable methods for tea decaffeination, but teas decaffeinated with these methods are not yet available, prob-

133

ably because this method is not as cost-effective for tea as it is for coffee, and because demand for these products is low. In any event, given our discussion of tea's fluoride content, the unavailability of solvent-free decaffeinated tea may be for the best in that it reduces our fluoride intakes.

I sometimes happen upon a tea decaffeination method that you can use at home, and it consists of steeping the tea you are making for one minute in hot water, discarding the water, and brewing a new cup of tea that you will drink from the already used teabag. The idea is that a significant amount of the caffeine is released during the first minute, but enough flavor remains for an enjoyable beverage.

This method will not yield a completely decaffeinated tea nor a strong tasting tea, but you can give it a try if it appeals to you and fits into your schedule. Since there is some flavor loss with decaffeination in general for both tea and coffee, you may find the beverages below to be more flavorful and therefore more helpful in your decaffeination process.

Coffee Substitutes

Although the original American coffee substitute Postum is dead, possibly awaiting revival, there are a number of other coffee substitutes on the market, including Cafix, Pero, Roma, and Teeccino. Coffee substitutes are usually made from an herb or grain such as wheat, rye, barley, or chicory. The earliest popular coffee substitutes contained chicory, which is a form of endive.

During the Napoleonic era, the French became accustomed to chicory as a coffee substitute when real coffee was not available during Napoleon's Continental Blockade. When coffee was once more available in France, the French began the tradition of adding chicory to their coffee, apparently because they had grown accustomed to the herb's taste. The Creole French have continued in this tradition, and the local New Orleans coffee is a blend of coffee and chicory. Interestingly, chicory also became popular in the southern United States during the Civil War when the Union cut off the flow of coffee to the Confederacy via the Union Naval Blockade. So it seems that throughout its history as a coffee substitute, blockades have helped chicory gain favor.

Teeccino has taken the coffee substitute a step further by offering herbal coffee, which rather than being an instant coffee substitute, is brewed just like coffee. Herbal coffee contains a mix of grains, herbs, and fruits, depending on the flavor. This combination of ingredients and the brewing method provide for a different taste experience than the usual one-ingredient instant substitutes. Teeccino also provides an on-the-go version of its product in "tee-bag" form.

My first experience with Teeccino was with the tee-bags and I was impressed by the complexity of both the flavor and aroma. It makes for a hearty brew that you may enjoy when weaning yourself off of coffee. My favorite flavors are Java, Chocolaté, and Original. If you want to preserve your caffeine ritual by replacing your caffeinated beverage, I suggest you experiment with a few of the above products to see which you like best.

A Soda Substitute

Beyond the caffeine-free sodas that you can find at the supermarket, you can also start to make your own soda-type drink that is healthier and just as tasty. I make my own "soda" on occasion and it gives me more energy than the caffeinated kind. And it is the lasting, healthy kind of energy that burns cleanly and does not result in a crash. To make it, I mix one part water, one part club soda or seltzer, and one part fruit juice.

I typically use a citrus juice such as grapefruit or orange, but I also enjoy this beverage with pomegranate and cranberry juice, and you can experiment with a number of juices to see which you like best. This soda substitute is not free of sugar, but it has far less sugar than the soda that you can buy at the store and it works well both for providing energy and for weaning you off the store-bought stuff.

Depending on the juices that you choose, you will also be getting some healthy antioxidants in your new drink. Begin to work this substitute into your regular schedule of soda consumption, replacing your regular soda, and try to gradually wean yourself off of soda, and the substitute, altogether.

You can also try plain and flavored seltzers, which provide a little flavor and no calories whatsoever. I drink these on occasion when I am trying to cut back on my energy intake and I find them to be more filling than water, perhaps due to the bit of flavor and the carbonation. Flavored seltzers are a wonderful replacement for sugary sodas, and you can try these beverages with a slice of lime or lemon for added variety.

You can also make your own seltzer flavors by making a concentrated herbal tea and mixing it with plain seltzer (more on herbal teas below). Reducing your fructose intake by eliminating soda and sugary caffeinated beverages from your diet may be all that you need to do to become lean, or it will at least be a large step toward leanness, by both reducing your overall energy intake and by helping you feel full through increased leptin sensitivity.

Herbal Teas

Herbal tea is the most logical substitute for black and green tea. For thousands of years, people have been making teas from fruits, berries, leaves, roots, bark, twigs, shoots, and even pine needles. In comparison, the brewing and consumption of caffeinated beverages has a much shorter history. I'll describe some of my favorite herbal teas, but keep in mind that my list is in no way exhaustive.

I recommend trying a sample pack of assorted herbal teas so that you can discover which ones you like best. The large variety of herbal teas has a corresponding large variety of flavors. There truly is something for everyone, and you will likely find yourself having a great time exploring these new flavors. Celestial Seasonings makes a sampler pack called the Herb Tea Sampler, and I recommend you try this or a similar sampler pack to see which herbal teas you enjoy the most.

Peppermint

Peppermint is a hybrid mint native to Europe, the cross between watermint and spearmint. Humans have consumed peppermint for thousands of years, both as a tasty beverage and as a treatment for various health problems. The active ingredient in peppermint is menthol. This herb has received attention recently as a weight loss aid, supposedly being used by stars such as Victoria Beckham and Cheryl Cole to achieve fast weight loss.

Allegedly these two celebrities drink peppermint tea while refraining from food as part of a fast. All of that aside, the tea tastes great! Peppermint tea has always had a place in my household and has a history of use in my family as a digestive aid. It also tastes good combined with other herbal teas, and if you combine peppermint with its parent plant spearmint, you get doublemint tea, just like the gum.

Ginger

Ginger is a tuber native to Southeast Asia that is consumed as a food, spice, and medicine. Ginger can be made into a tea by stewing the raw tuber in boiling water, or by brewing commercially available ginger tea bags. Lemon is commonly added to ginger tea to enhance its flavor. Ginger is often used as a digestive aid and to relieve motion sickness and nausea. Ginger ale, ginger beer, and ginger water have been used throughout the world as digestive aids. Ginger tea has also been used in folk medicine as an immune system stimulant to prevent and treat colds and flu. Ginger tea is spicy, and you can brew it strong or weak depending on your preferences.

Rooibos

One of my favorite caffeine-free beverages that I enjoy both hot and cold is rooibos tea, also known as red bush tea and red tea. The rooibos plant is native to South Africa, and the teas come in red and green varieties, with red being oxidized and green non-oxidized. I prefer the red tea, which is more flavorful than the green version due to the effects of oxidation. The flavor of red rooibos tea comes very close to that of black tea. That being said, green rooibos tea has more of a grassy flavor which many people find pleasing, so you may want to try both.

Rooibos tea is commonly taken with a slice of lemon and some sugar much like black tea, and the method of preparation is the same. Some South African cafés serve rooibos espressos, lattés and cappuccinos, which I hope to try one day. I make my own iced version of the tea in the summer that is delicious.

Sweet Herbal Tea

I spent some time in the South and I developed a liking for sweet tea. The great thing about sweet tea when compared to the tea that Northerners drink is that it is brewed with the sugar in it. More precisely, the sugar is added before the tea has a chance to get cold, and this results in more of the sugar being dissolved in the tea. I took it a step further when I used to make my own sweet tea by putting tea, water, and sugar on a low boil for a few minutes or until it reduced enough for me to add ice and colder water. It always turned out wonderfully.

I tried to do the same thing with rooibos tea and the result was substantially the same! Although the flavor is less tannic, making it differ from black tea, I find sweet rooibos tea to be a pleasing alternative. If you do not want to boil the tea and sugar mixture, just make sure that when you pour hot water over the tea that the sugar is already in place. Then cool, add ice, and enjoy! You can use the same strategy with many of the other drinks in this section; just make sure that if you are adding ice and cold water that you make your original infusion more concentrated to allow for the dilution with the ice and cold water. Sweet rooibos tea is not sugar-free, so don't go overboard.

Cinnamon

Cinnamon is the bark of a small evergreen tree native to Sri Lanka, and it has been used as a spice for flavoring and preservation purposes for centuries. If you enjoy the taste of cinnamon you can try some of the cinnamon teas on

139

the market or you can simply add cinnamon to the other beverages in this chapter. An added benefit of using cinnamon in teas and in food is that it helps to lower blood sugar by enhancing your body's insulin sensitivity. In this way cinnamon can be another effective tool for combating high insulin levels, and thereby the cravings and resultant overeating that accompany both insulin resistance and low blood sugar spells.

Chamomile

Chamomile is the daisy-like, national flower of Russia. Chamomile has been used for centuries for a variety of ailments and for its mild sedative properties that many people find helpful both for stress relief and as a sleep aid. Although this might not be a good replacement for your morning cup of coffee since it can make you a little too relaxed to work, I include it because it can be quite soothing in the evening or even during the day when you feel overcome by life.

Adaptogen Herbs

Adaptogen herbs are herbs that help the body cope with stress, and some people find these to be helpful when they are coming off of caffeine or facing any one of life's stressors. These herbs work by stimulating the immune system, and while I do not use any of them on a regular basis, I find that they do help me on occasion. The adaptogen herbs include Siberian ginseng, Panax ginseng, echinacea, astragalus, reishi mushrooms, and schizandra.

If you look at some of the herbal teas on the market, it is easy to find a few that have ginseng or echinacea added to them, so you can try one of the herbs in this category as part of a commercially prepared blend and see what its effects are for you.

Fruit teas

Fruit teas are brewed from fruits such as oranges, apples, and various berries. There are a number of commercially available fruit teas and you can also brew your own at home from fresh and dried fruit. Celestial Seasonings makes a sampler pack called the Fruit Tea Sampler which I have tried and enjoy very much, so I recommend that you give that or a similar sampler pack a try.

This is a good option if you are trying to avoid sugar because the tea bags will not contain any sugar, whereas if you brew your own fruit tea from fresh and dried fruit you will inevitably be consuming the sugar and calories from the fruit itself. Fruit teas are perfect for brewing, cooling, and adding ice and seltzer to, thereby creating your own fruit-flavored, caffeine-free, zero calorie sodas.

I also like some of the herbal tea blends such as Twinings' Herbal Unwind, which is a blend of orange peel, cinnamon, peppermint, ginger, and hibiscus. There are many different herbal blends that you can get in tea bags, and of course you can steal the recipes on the box and make your own. I find the blends that have some citrus and some spice to be very refreshing, both as hot beverages in the winter and with ice in the summer.

Try out a sample pack of assorted herbal teas and herbal tea blends so that you can discover which ones you like best. There is a large variety of herbal teas with a corresponding variety of flavors. There truly is something for everyone, and you might find yourself having a great time exploring these new flavors.

Water

Water is always a viable beverage option, underrated as it is, and those of us who prefer simplicity may choose to use water as our main caffeine-free beverage. Should you become bored with this wonderful resource, however, go ahead and try one of the beverages suggested above.

This completes our discussion of replacement beverages, and now we'll move on to some dietary and lifestyle strategies that will help to make your transition to a reduced or nonexistent caffeine intake much easier.

Mood Support

If you're used to caffeine's "pick-me-up" effect, then reducing your caffeine consumption can have a negative impact on your mood. Now that you're no longer stimulating serotonin release via caffeine intake, you'll have to find a way to maintain a healthy, happiness-promoting serotonin level in other ways. Fortunately, there are some simple lifestyle changes that you can implement (in addition to your fruit and vegetable rich diet) to maintain your positive mood.

While a number of health and nutrition experts recommend supplements for mood support, I am not a big believer in the advantages of supplements over whole, fresh foods, so I do not list these supplements here. If that is something that interests you, then a simple internet search for natural supplements for mood support should point you in the right direction.

Exercise, exposure to bright light, and fish oil consumption are natural ways to increase serotonin levels without resorting to caffeine.[204] Exercise also promotes the production of endorphins, which help contribute to feelings of well-being and can help to replace your caffeine highs. If you eat small, oily fish once or twice a week, exercise regularly, and get regular sun exposure, you will be doing a lot to get a natural serotonin boost without caffeine. Prozac, which raises serotonin levels, is one of the most commonly prescribed medications in the United States. Let diet and exercise raise your serotonin levels naturally when possible, rather than turning to prescription drugs.

Exercise

Before you begin any exercise program, make sure that you receive clearance from your physician that you are healthy enough to do so. You should try to make exercise a regular part of your life, so that you can experience higher levels of well-being through serotonin release, for muscle maintenance, for exercise's metabolic effects, and as a direct way of increasing your energy expenditure. You burn calories directly when you exercise, because your muscles, heart, lungs, and other organs all require energy to perform physical exercise. When you finish exercising, your heart rate and your rate of breathing take some time to resume their resting rates, so you continue to burn calories at a higher rate after exercise.

This is sometimes called the after-burn effect of exercise, or post-exercise oxygen consumption. In addition to the increased energy expenditure during and after exercise, you also improve your thyroid function and help to maintain your muscle mass by exercising, both of which can increase your daily resting energy expenditure. Both aerobic and resistance exercise will also help sensitize your muscles to insulin's action, helping avoid or improve any issues with insulin resistance, insulin-induced overeating, and low blood sugar-induced overeating. I know what you're thinking, it seems that exercise's list of benefits are endless.

What kind of exercise is best to achieve the maximum results as far as burning fat? Both cardiovascular and resistance training should be a part of your regular exercise regimen, but before we reach the specifics of your new training routine, let's briefly discuss one of the latest exercise fads.

It is currently the fashion in the fitness community to proclaim that aerobic exercise is useless for weight loss. The opponents of aerobic exercise claim that resistance exercise is better for weight loss, and sometimes go so far as to say that running, biking, and swimming cause fat gain. I think this reaction is due in part to the fact that most people despise cardiovascular exercise, and will find ways to rationalize avoiding it.

Whether aerobic exercise or resistance exercise is better for your personal fat loss depends on a large number of factors, including duration of exercise, exercise intensity, overeating behaviors associated with each type of exercise, and so forth. If you are concerned about overeating after you exercise, I have good news. There is no evidence that small amounts of exercise produce compensatory increases in energy intake in individuals who are mostly sedentary.[205]

So if you're new to exercise, you don't have to worry about it making you very hungry. People have different appetite responses to exercise. Some feel hungrier after exercise, and others feel less hungry. That aside, which type of exercise to do should not be an either/or proposition. Both aerobic and resistance exercise have their place in an exercise program!

I speak from experience as a former athlete and current sports enthusiast, and from the experience of countless trainers and athletes with whom I've had the pleasure of training. I've omitted aerobic exercise for months at a time to try out resistance-only training routines. I used high-intensity methods, including circuit training, and this did not translate well to cardiovascular fitness when I started running and swimming again. In fact, my aerobic capacity had decreased with the omission of aerobic exercise. And no, I did not become fat as a result of doing aerobic exercise. I know it seems obvious, but the value of aerobic exercise has somehow become a hotly contested issue in the fitness community.

Now I'm not recommending that you become a marathon runner, just that you consider doing 1-2 hours of aerobic exercise per week as a starting point, distributed among 20-30 minute sessions, or sessions of a different length that suit you based on your lifestyle, schedule, and fitness level. And this should be aerobic exercise that you enjoy, so that you don't become a member of the "aerobic exercise is fattening" cult.

You can start by walking or playing a sport that you like. When I don't feel up to running due to the heat or other reasons, I walk with my headphones and portable mp3 player and listen to music or audiobooks. If you have some nice scenery in your area, you can walk, hike, and run on trails. I often walk and run on the boardwalk and beach where I live, and I find that exercising outdoors is much more stimulating than exercising indoors. Walking and running on a treadmill, while staring at the wall, will not a lover of aerobic exercise make.

Scenery isn't the only factor in your exercise regimen that makes for effective, enjoyable training that you can maintain as part of your routine for the long-term. Having good company in the form of a motivated training partner can be the difference between an exercise schedule that you enjoy and one that you dread. Find an exercise partner or group to walk, run, or play sports with, and you will enjoy your exercise routine even more while reaping all of its benefits.

Then again, you may prefer to exercise in solitude, using your exercise time for meditative personal reflection. If you are just starting out, aim for at least 20 minutes of aerobic activity 3-4 times a week and you can increase this level of activity as you become more fit and you can also make adjustments based on how quickly you are achieving your weight loss goals. If you are walking two miles a day three times a week and you find that this is easy and want to reach your healthy weight faster, by all means walk on the other days too, if your schedule and energy levels allow for it.

Once you've made cardiovascular exercise a regular part of your life, you should begin to add some resistance training to your routine so that you can put on some lean weight and add to your body's fat-burning muscle mass. Cardiovascular exercise will also help put some muscle on your frame, especially if you were not previously physically active, but resistance exercise is a must if you want to maximize your fat-burning body mass.

Once you are comfortable with your new exercise regimen and your doctor believes you are fit enough, start on a basic resistance training routine. Start slow, with exercises that emphasize a large number of muscle groups. This is not an exercise book and I don't want to turn it into one, but I will share my favorite muscle-building exercises that I believe most people would benefit from.

At some points in my life I have just about lived in the gym, and I admit that I am a bit of a fitness freak. With that in mind, if you asked me to pick the absolute best exercises for muscle building, I would say pull-ups and lunges. Those are the exercises that will give you the most results for the time you put in. What is excellent about these exercises is that they work a lot of muscles at the same time, and if you use dumbbells for the lunges, these two exercises will not put much compressive force on your spine, so if done correctly they should not aggravate any existing or potential back problems. I know what you're thinking, you can't do any pull-ups. Well, it's never too late to learn. Everyone should be able to do at least five bodyweight pull-ups without collapsing in a heap afterwards, women too.

The best way to learn to do a pull-up if you can not do one is not by using the assisted pull-up machine, which is of course what most people do and never learn to do unassisted pull-ups. The best way to start doing pull-ups is to do negative pull-ups. All that means is that you jump or use something to stand on to get yourself into the top of a pull up position, and then lower yourself as slowly as you can.

If you work these into your exercise regimen, you will be doing real pull-ups before long. In addition, if you have access to a gym, the lat pulldown machine will help you with your pull-up strength. When you do finally get it, it will feel like a great victory. Once you incorporate pull-ups or the lat pulldown and lunges into your routine, you can add a basic pressing movement, such as the dumbbell press, which is another excellent movement in that it has limited injury potential and works multiple muscle groups at the same time.

Please look up proper exercise form and consult with a physician before attempting these exercises. **www.exrx.net**, and **www.tmuscle.com** are both excellent resources, but pictures often can not do what a trainer or workout partner can do to correct your technique. You may benefit from hiring a trainer to show you proper exercise technique, or you can learn proper technique on your own through the large number of online muscle-building resources. There are also some very good books on muscle building that you can browse at the library and bookstores before deciding which you would like to purchase.

Falling off the Wagon

While you are decaffeinating, cheating is likely, and per-haps inevitable. You may fall off of the caffeine-free wagon from time to time, and you may choose to drink some coffee with dessert on occasion and there is nothing wrong with that. There's no need to feel shame or guilt when and if you relapse, it's a normal part of changing your routine. If you do catch yourself cheating on this plan, chances are you have reduced your consumption of caffeine too quickly, or not quickly enough, depending on whether you are trying gradual reduction or quitting cold turkey. Consider that the opposite of the method you are currently using might work better for you if you are having difficulties.

So if you are trying to quit cold turkey and you are having problems, try the gradual reduction method and see if that works better for you. If you are trying the gradual reduction method and you are having problems, try quitting cold tur-key and see if that works better for you. What you should also try to do is to make sure that if and when you do cheat, you do so in reducing degrees of severity. In other words, each time you cheat, make sure that you cheat less than the previous time. Furthermore, if you are going to cheat to get the caffeine high that you miss, try to do so in accordance with the strategies outlined in the next chapter, Optimal Caffeine Use.

Other Health Issues

Caffeine contributes to a number of health problems be-sides weight gain and the problems that weight gain brings with it. These health issues are beyond the scope of this book, as we are interested primarily in caffeine's contribu-tion to the obesity and weight gain epidemic. For those who are interested however, I will describe the negative health

148

effects that I experience from indulging too freely in caffeinated beverages. The most common caffeine side effect for me is cold hands and feet, due to reduced peripheral circulation. This reduction in circulation is another part of the stress response that we discussed in Chapter 3, Caffeine and Cortisol.

It is interesting to note here that caffeine consumption also reduces circulation to the brain, and this decreased circulation is part of the reason for the withdrawal headaches that come with missing a dose of caffeine. When the body eliminates enough caffeine to begin to resume normal, healthy blood flow to the brain, this larger blood flow is what causes the caffeine withdrawal headache with which we are all painfully familiar.

The other caffeine side effects that I commonly experience are joint pain, increased thirst, increased stress, and increased irritability. Other common side effects of caffeine include insomnia, nervousness, restlessness, agitation, gastric irritation, nausea, vomiting, fast heartbeat, arrhythmias, increased respiratory rate, muscle spasms, ringing in the ears, headache, delirium, and convulsions.[206]

For more information on the negative health effects of caffeine consumption, please read Stephen Cherniske's *Caffeine Blues*, which is an excellent synthesis of caffeine's various negative health consequences beyond weight gain and obesity. If you follow the program in this chapter and reduce or eliminate your caffeine intake, you may find that your health improves in a number of surprising ways apart from weight loss.

Summary

Your two options for reducing or eliminating your caffeine consumption are gradually reducing your intake and quitting caffeine cold turkey. Different people will have varying levels of success with each of these methods. Some will find it easier to gradually taper their caffeine intakes, while others will find it easier to quit cold turkey. Replacement beverages are helpful in reducing or eliminating your caffeine intake because they allow you to keep some parts of your caffeine-drinking ritual intact.

Replacement beverages include the caffeine-free and decaffeinated versions of your favorite beverages, as well as coffee substitutes, herbal teas, fruit teas, seltzer, and water. My favorite herbal teas that I recommend you try are rooibos, peppermint, chamomile, ginger, and cinnamon. Don't get discouraged if you find yourself turning back to caffeine once in a while in your efforts to reduce your consumption. You will be successful over time.

The two lifestyle aids detailed in this chapter are those of mood support and exercise. For mood-enhancing effects that you will no longer be getting from caffeine, turn to exercise, oily fish consumption, and exposure to sunlight. For the energy expenditure and metabolic benefits of exercise, I recommend that you slowly incorporate both cardiovascular and resistance training into your schedule.

In the next chapter, we'll explore how you can continue to consume caffeine while blunting its fattening effects. The mood support and exercise lifestyle aids described in this chapter should be used as part of the optimal caffeine use strategy described in the next chapter. These lifestyle aids will help keep the negative effects of caffeine consumption under some control.

CHAPTER 8
OPTIMAL CAFFEINE USE

The voodoo priest and all his powders were as nothing compared to espresso, cappuccino, and mocha, which are stronger than all the religions of the world combined, and perhaps stronger than the human soul itself.

-Mark Helprin, *Memoir from Antproof Case* (1995)

This chapter is a necessity, as most people will never give up caffeine. I myself enjoy some coffee or chocolate once in a while. Caffeine is so omnipresent that its at least sporadic consumption may be inevitable. And if caffeine is in fact stronger than the human soul, we must have a plan to deal with it. With that in mind, I put this chapter together so that those of us who choose to consume caffeine regularly or on occasion can do so while minimizing its fattening effects.

Please follow the recommendations in the previous chapter in the Mood Support and Exercise sections if caffeine is to remain a part of your diet. By doing so, you will already be accomplishing much in counteracting caffeine's effects in increasing your energy intake and lowering your energy expenditure.

Tin Foil Hats

Conspiracy theorists sometimes suggest that food manufacturers put caffeine and chocolate in their food products
to make these products addictive, noting that the FDA
does not require the labeling of caffeine content, so that
we would not know about the presence of hidden caffeine.
This would be beneficial for sales of the caffeine-containing
products, and so it would be advantageous for food manufacturers to employ any kind of strategy that makes their
food products addictive.

Whether or not food manufacturers purposely do this and
other conspiracy theories aside, the fact remains that many
caffeine and chocolate-containing foods contain a lot of
calories, and contribute to weight gain. Since almost all
people are regular consumers of caffeine and chocolate,
they are also exposed to the side calories present along with
caffeine and cocoa. If we are to reduce our overall calorie
intakes while retaining our consumption of caffeine and
chocolate, we must reduce or eliminate these side calories.
The natural strategy is to adopt a method of low calorie caffeine use.

Low Calorie Caffeine Use

If we are to continue with caffeine as a regular part of our
weight loss diets, we must be careful to consume caffeine
in a way that limits all of the side calories that come with
it. First, that means that if we are used to a certain caffeine
ritual, we must reevaluate this ritual and its impact on our
diet. If we regularly complement our cup of coffee with a
big fatty and sugary muffin or other pastry, we can improve
this ritual by eliminating the pastry and substituting half a
banana.

From there, we can start to reduce the amount of cream and sugar that we take in the coffee, gradually phasing it out. Finally, we can phase out the banana as well. What we are left with is a cup of black coffee, with almost no calories. (An average cup of coffee without sugar or cream weighs in at approximately 5 calories, an amount not worth worrying about.)

Ideally, when taking caffeine, we should strive to do so without any side calories. Your low calorie caffeine beverage options include coffee without cream or sugar, teas without cream or sugar, maté without cream or sugar, and cocoa without cream or sugar. Since our main draw to these substances is the caffeine and theobromine, those are all that we need to get our fix. It is not the sugar and cream that our bodies are addicted to in these beverages, but the caffeine.

So by satisfying our addiction to caffeine without the additional calories, and especially without all the fructose, we may blunt at least the addiction-driven overeating that accompanies caffeine consumption. The great thing is that by cutting out the side calories in your caffeinated beverages or eliminating these beverages altogether, you cut back on fructose. In doing so, not only do you reduce your calorie intake directly, but you also help re-sensitize your body to leptin, so you feel more full while simultaneously reducing your energy intake!

If you are in the habit of buying or making very sugary and creamy coffee and tea, then once you switch to taking your coffee and tea all by itself, you'll have cut out 300 or more calories from your daily routine. Even if switching to black coffee cuts only 100-200 calories from your daily intake, this will make a big difference over time to your body composition. If you drink multiple high-calorie caffeinated beverages throughout the day, then eliminating the side calories will make an even larger difference to your energy intake. Cutting out these side calories will reduce your energy intake such that 1) you begin to lose weight; or 2) you stop gaining weight; or 3) your rate of weight gain slows.

All of these effects are desirable if you are trying to improve your body composition by reducing your body fat. The average American adult, who gains 1-2 pounds per year, has an approximate positive energy balance of just 10-50 calories per day.[207] This does not take into account binge eating, but it demonstrates that a small daily calorie reduction can have a large impact if it is carried out in the long-term. A small step, such as removing the sugar and cream from your coffee, can have a large impact on your weight over the space of months and years.

What about soda? Unfortunately, if you are a soda lover, the only recommendation I can make regarding this beverage is that you phase it out gradually or reduce it to levels at which you can successfully maintain a lean physique. While a variety of artificially sweetened low-calorie sodas exist, I can not in good faith recommend these to anyone, and the same goes for any energy drinks or other foods that are artificially sweetened. From a pure calorie balance perspective, they seem to be alright at first glance, but they actually disrupt the body's ability to gauge satiety, as we discussed in Chapter 5, Addiction-Driven Overeating.

Given that aspartame and other artificial sweeteners are associated with behavioral and neurological problems, and who knows what other unknown health problems, I stay away from these beverages. While I know many people who drink these beverages regularly and stay relatively lean, I personally must have an intolerance to aspartame, as I can drink regular soda and feel fine, but artificially sweetened soda makes me ill for hours. I get severe headaches from aspartame, as well as nausea and on two occasions vomiting. From these experiences I have learned to stay away from this substance and perhaps my body's reaction is a good thing, keeping me away from this new chemical sweetener.

A no-calorie sweetener that I do use sometimes and do not experience negative side effects from is stevia. Stevia is an herb with sweet leaves that grows in tropical and subtropical regions. This herb is 300 times sweeter than sugar, and contains virtually no calories. The native peoples of South America have used stevia as a sweetener for centuries, with no apparent side effects. There is some preliminary evidence that stevia may improve insulin sensitivity, and this coincides with its use in South America as a traditional herbal treatment for type 2 diabetes, so stevia may even help combat insulin-induced overeating.

Stevia has been the subject of some controversy in the United States due to the FDA's 1991 determination that the herb was unsafe as a food additive. This determination was controversial because under the FDA's guidelines, stevia should have been labeled safe, as long as it was a natural substance that had been used before 1958 with no reported side effects, and was being used in the same way after 1958 (stevia satisfied these criteria). Stevia consumers responded with allegations that the FDA gave stevia an unsafe designation in order to protect the domestic artificial sweetener industries. In 1995 the FDA permitted the use of stevia as a dietary supplement, while retaining its unsafe designation as a food additive.

In 2008, the FDA approved the new sweeteners Truvia and PureVia as safe. Both of these sweeteners are derivatives of stevia. Truvia was developed by the Coca-Cola Company, and PureVia was developed by PepsiCo. Now that the soft drink giants are in the stevia game, the FDA has no problem going along. Stevia has made a lot of progress in the marketplace recently; just the other day I saw stevia packets for sale in a Duane Reade in New York City under the Duane Reade brand. Truvia products include Vitaminwater Zero, Sprite Green, vitaminwater 10, Minute Maid Enhanced Pomegranate Flavored Tea, Dippin' Dots, Blue Sky Free Soda, True Lemon Naturally Sweet, All Sport Naturally Zero, Odwalla Mojito Mambo, and Odwalla Pomegranate Strawberry. PureVia products include Sobe Lifewater Black and Blue Berry, and Sobe Lifewater Fuji Apple Pear Water. Maybe you've already had these sweeteners without even knowing it.

I use stevia in moderation to flavor herbal teas and coffees and I have not experienced any ill effects from it. As for its taste, the sweet taste it provides differs from that of sugar. I find that it goes better with herbal tea than with coffee or coffee substitutes, but tastes differ. If you choose to use this herb as a sweetener you can experiment with how much you like to use and what brands you prefer. I recently purchased some stevia extract with vanilla in it, and I find this extra flavor to be pleasant, so that is another stevia option with a slightly different taste that you can try out. Don't forget to stir after you add stevia to your beverage, as it has a tendency to sink straight to the bottom before dissolving.

Keep in mind that artificial sweeteners and stevia both cause a slight insulin response due to their sweet taste even though they are virtually carbohydrate free. Their sweet taste prompts the body to expect sugar and so insulin rises before blood glucose levels have gone up. I include this note because it is interesting that the body has this anticipatory response, but I don't think we should obsess about it. Please also note that while stevia is a better alternative sweetener than artificial sweeteners, it may still have the same effect as artificial sweeteners in reducing your body's ability to gauge caloric intake, so use in moderation.

Cortisol Control

In order to minimize caffeine's effects on your cortisol levels, one of the best things you can do is to try to cut back on your caffeine consumption at times when you are, or expect to be, experiencing high levels of stress. This may not be feasible for those of us with stress-filled and highly demanding jobs, so you will need to focus on dietary and lifestyle support in order to keep caffeine from adding to your existing stress levels. The dietary support strategy was discussed in Chapter 3, Caffeine and Cortisol.

If you recall, the nutritional support for reducing your cortisol levels comes down to including a variety of fresh fruits and vegetables in your diet on a regular basis, so you can maintain healthy levels of cortisol-reducing vitamin C. By keeping your cortisol levels from getting completely out of control, these strategies will help you reduce the cortisol-induced overeating and muscle breakdown resulting from caffeine consumption.

Insulin Control

In order to minimize caffeine's effects on your insulin levels, you will need to think about the timing of your caffeine consumption. This is in addition to the removal of sugar from your caffeinated beverages. To keep your levels of blood sugar and insulin stable while consuming caffeine, you must try to take caffeine separately from other foods, especially from carbohydrate-rich foods. If you plan on having a meal that is high in carbohydrates for lunch, for example, then try to have your caffeine a few hours before lunch.

This is tough to do if you are going to have caffeine several times throughout the day, and may require a diet that is low in carbohydrates in order for you to avoid the caffeine-induced wild blood sugar and insulin fluctuations that can lead to overeating. You can also try adding cinnamon to your coffee and see if you enjoy the taste. Cinnamon will help a little with regulating your insulin and blood sugar levels and will also add some more flavor to your coffee.

For further improving your insulin sensitivity while you consume caffeinated foods and beverages, try to exercise and expose yourself to small amounts of sunlight regularly. It is interesting that less insulin resistance will provide your cells with more energy for exercise, and that more exercise lessens insulin resistance. It's no wonder that regular exercisers have more energy than the rest of us!

Best Sources

If you choose to continue consuming caffeine, where should you get it from? Which sources are the best in terms of having the fewest negative effects for your resting energy expenditure? Now that you've decided to take your caffeinated beverages without any side calories, let's go over which caffeinated beverages to favor.

First, due to the fluoride content of teas, practice moderation when consuming green and black teas unless you know that the teas you drink are low in fluoride. At this point I have not found any brands of tea that monitor for fluoride content, so the best I can do is to recommend you practice moderation or avoid tea altogether. If you know or suspect that you have an underactive thyroid, stay away from green and black tea. You can get all of the antioxidant benefits of green and black tea from other plant sources, including fruits, vegetables, berries, and herbal teas.

Eliminating tea leaves coffee and cocoa as the only widely available caffeine sources that you can find without significant side calories and without artificial sweeteners. So to consume caffeine in an optimal way, have small amounts of coffee and cocoa without added sugar or cream, but perhaps with small amounts of stevia instead. If you do add sugar and/or cream, do so in moderation and avoid making your cup of caffeine a meal.

If you have trouble staying away from chocolate, it is likely the unique theobromine-caffeine cocktail that you crave. Your best strategy is to get this special fix from a concentrated source such as pure cocoa that you can brew yourself, or from small amounts of dark chocolate, rather than trying to get your theobromine fix from a diluted high calorie source such as chocolate chip cookies or chocolate ice cream.

To get the same amount of theobromine in two cups of low calorie brewed cocoa, you may have to eat several packages of calorie-filled Oreos, or several pints of chocolate ice cream. Stay away from diluted chocolate sources such as these and strive to take chocolate the way the Maya and Aztec originally took it – in water, without sugar, thickly mixed and with some pepper or berries for flavor.

You can even mimic the ancient way of taking chocolate exactly, and take your bitter cup of cocoa cold, rather than hot. Who knows, perhaps you will fall in love with this low calorie beverage. I have no doubt that it would be very popular today if it were not for the extreme abundance of junk foods and sweeteners that have turned us off to taking any beverages in unsweetened form.

Do caffeine pills fit into an optimal caffeine use plan? It seems that they do because they offer a standardized dose of caffeine without any additional calories. Pills may be worthy of your consideration, but I personally avoid them because if I am going to have caffeine, I want to have it in a more enjoyable, more antioxidant-rich form than a pill. If you choose to use pills, be careful of the dose you take and keep in mind that 100 mg of caffeine is the amount usually found in one cup of coffee. People have died from overdosing on caffeine pills.

What's Missing?

With the exception of your caffeinated foods and beverages and their timing, I'm not asking you to make many dietary modifications. Why not? Because if you follow the strategies in the Decaf Plan chapter and in this chapter, you will reduce your energy intake and simultaneously increase your energy expenditure, without having to think very much about the rest of your food intake. The above steps will put you in negative calorie balance, or at least closer to it than you were previously.

After you've manipulated your caffeine intake, you'll find that you can eat less because much of your hunger is gone, and your recovering metabolism will take care of at least some of the fat loss for you. For me, whenever I stopped my caffeine intake, my appetite down-regulated itself automatically, I just wasn't as hungry as I had been while consuming caffeine. Combine that with your now faster resting energy expenditure and new exercise routine, and the weight loss will take care of itself.

I don't believe in giving people restrictive food lists, because everyone's tastes and preferences differ. We are all different, and there is not a perfect universal diet. As you've probably gathered from the rest of this book, if you back me into a corner and make me give you specific food advice, I would just say eat a variety of whole fresh foods that you enjoy, and if you don't enjoy whole fresh foods, try to incorporate them into your diet gradually (or all at once if that suits you) until you find your tastes changing, and your tastes will change if you coax them. But I don't want to give you specific food advice beyond my advice regarding caffeine.

People who are naturally lean usually don't diet, and they don't think about dieting. They have healthy appetite regulation, healthy resting metabolisms, and are physically active, and the leanness takes care of itself. By following my caffeine recommendations, you can restore your healthy appetite regulation and resting metabolism, and become "naturally" lean by letting your body take care of itself. I hope you achieve lasting leanness and its associated health benefits.

Summary

If you will continue to keep caffeine in your diet, strive to get your fix from low calorie sources, as you will have to grapple with cortisol-induced and insulin-induced hunger and overeating. Stick to beverages to which you do not add cream or sugar. In order to minimize caffeine's negative effects on your stress and cortisol levels, maintain a healthy intake of fruits and vegetables and try to reduce your caffeine consumption in times of stress. In order to minimize caffeine's negative effects on your insulin system, make sure you take your caffeinated beverage of choice without sugar, and separate in time from carbohydrate-rich foods and meals.

The best sources of caffeine are coffee, hot cocoa, and low fluoride teas if you can find them. If you know or suspect that you have an underactive thyroid, you may benefit from moderating or eliminating tea as a dietary caffeine source.

By adjusting your caffeine intake as described in this chapter and by following the Mood Support and Exercise recommendations in the previous chapter, you can improve your body composition while retaining your caffeine consumption. If you choose to reduce or eliminate your caffeine consumption in accordance with the previous chapter, your results will be even better.

For optimal caffeine use, I am not asking you to modify your energy intake in any other ways besides eliminating side calories and maintaining your fruit and vegetable consumption. The elimination of these side calories will reduce your energy intake and decrease your tendency to overeat by reducing your fructose intake. The reduction in fructose intake will also decrease your tendency to store fat centrally, improving the proportions of your body. That's it! Now let's move on to that mind-blowing, life-changing conclusion that I promised you at the beginning of the book.

CHAPTER 9
LASTING LEANNESS

Be careful about reading health books. You may die of a misprint.

-Mark Twain

In the 18th century, King Gustav III of Sweden was convinced that coffee and tea were poisons and set out to prove it. He forced one convicted murderer to drink coffee every day, and another convicted murderer to drink tea every day. Both murderers outlived Gustav III, the tea drinker being the first to die at the age of 83.[208]

Gustav III was not alone. For centuries, starting as soon as caffeine took off as a popular stimulant throughout the world, the opponents of caffeine have been threatening caffeine consumers with all kinds of diseases.[209] I do not see myself as an opponent of caffeine use per se, but as a proponent of its proper and responsible use, as well as its reduction or even elimination in the diets of those who are trying to lose weight. As wondrous as caffeine may be as a stimulant, it is not a suitable addition to a weight loss diet.

Caffeine the Modernizer

One of the central arguments made by Bennett Weinberg and Bonnie Bealer, the authors of *The World of Caffeine,* is that the modern world was made possible by the contemporaneous proliferation of beverage caffeine and timekeeping devices, because caffeine allows people to work on a set schedule.[210] In *Uncommon Grounds,* Mark Pendergrast echoes this argument and maintains that coffee's popularity to some degree sustained the Industrial Revolution.[211]

I agree to a large extent, but we must also consider that a major stimulus for progress in this time period was not so much caffeine itself, but caffeine as a replacement for alcohol. Before caffeine appeared on the scene, much of Europe was drunk from morning to night, and constant drunkenness does not a productive workforce make.

People love drugs, and caffeine supplanted much of the alcohol in the human diet. It is likely that modernization would have taken longer if we were sluggishly drunk at work, rather than high with the frenetic energy of caffeine. Today, caffeine is still an economic stimulant, driving many of our nation's best thinkers to improve our technology and infrastructure.

Interestingly, as our technology and infrastructure improve, the less we need to rely on our own bodies for movement and entertainment. We can drive rather than walk, and play soccer on the internet rather than on a real field. In much of the United States, walking is a thing of the past, and sports have taken a backseat to technology-driven entertainment that we enjoy while seated or lying down.

In our now sedentary lives, we regard caffeine-containing beverages as smart-drinks and energizers, turning to them when we need to stay up late for work or study, and when we need to be alert or simply awake for long periods of time.[212]

And though there is no doubt that caffeine is a productivity crutch for many, its necessity in this regard is questionable. Although most of us rely on caffeine for what we think is an energy boost, we are more often than not just using caffeine to relieve our withdrawal symptoms. Many people are productive without regular caffeine consumption, and living without caffeine is possible, as strange as this notion may seem to most of us.

Caffeine the Socializer

We now live in a café society, where the café plays a central role in much of our social activity.[213] The coffeehouse provides a place for friends and strangers to meet; an informal gathering place for social and intellectual discourse. Throughout history, the coffeehouse has served as a place for people to meet and discuss a large variety of matters, most notably politics. For this reason, a number of governments all over the world have tried to ban coffeehouses (houses of sedition) at many points in history.[214]

Efforts to ban coffee and the coffeehouse were usually unsuccessful, resulting in a black market for coffee and the rise of coffee speakeasies until the government realized that there was more money to be made in taxing coffee than in ineffectively banning it.[215] The governments' initial failure to capitalize on the coffee trade in many ways parallels the United States' reluctance to legalize and profit from marijuana. But that is neither here nor there.

Nowadays, the coffeehouse is less a place for political discussion, and more a place to do work and meet members of the opposite sex. In Finland, inviting a member of the opposite sex for coffee is so much a part of the courting ritual that ads for casual sex go in the form of ads for a "day-coffee companion."[216] We are not so different from Finland, as the shyly stammered phrase, "Want to get a cup of coffee?" is unequivocally a come-on.

It's great that coffeehouses provide such an effective environment for social discourse. But in a nation and world that is getting fatter by the cup, we need to reconsider the role of the coffeehouse and caffeine in terms of their impact on our waistlines. Coffeehouses do have caffeine-free and low calorie caffeinated drinks, and it is time that we begin to demand more of these alternative beverages if we are to continue frequenting coffeehouses while we strive to lose weight and stay lean.

Lasting Leanness

Close to 70% of American adults are overweight, and the incidence of obesity is rising. The rate of obesity is currently increasing at approximately one percent per year, and as yet this trend does not show any sign of slowing.[217] The obesity epidemic has not yet peaked, so its full implications may not be felt for some time. Many researchers are trying to pinpoint the change in the early 1980s that caused the rate of weight gain in the United States to increase so dramatically. Although some researchers point to the increasing use of high-fructose corn syrup as the single most important shift, it is likely that there were a number of changes that occurred simultaneously, that contributed to increasing our energy intakes and decreasing our energy expenditures.[218]

Large quantities of calorie-dense food are cheaply available, and are advertised heavily. Our physical activity has declined markedly. Most of us lead sedentary lives where we no longer need to be physically active. Some researchers estimate that we expend 1,500 less calories per day in physical activity than our predecessors two generations before.[219] That is a huge difference, and unfortunately most of us do not have the time to burn 1500 calories per day through exercise. Such a high level of physical activity is no longer practicable given our modern day lifestyles.

As I mentioned in the beginning of the book, there is disagreement among the researchers concerning whether increased food intake or decreased levels of physical activity play a greater role in the current obesity epidemic.[220] Some researchers argue that increased energy intake, rather than decreased energy expenditure, is the primary driver of the obesity epidemic.[221] Other researchers take the other side of this argument. I think it is safe to say that both increased food intake and decreased physical activity work together to make us fat.

There is also disagreement as to whether decreasing food intake or increasing physical activity is the best way of dealing with the obesity epidemic. Again, while both sides of the equation were important in making us fat, the solution is more complicated, because many of us have difficulty making time for exercise. As a result, solving the nation's weight problem requires individuals to take measures that are appropriate and specific to their own lifestyles, and that requires an understanding that energy balance is the key to weight loss.

We have discussed how caffeine contributes to overeating and increases energy intake through its effects on cortisol and insulin, and due to the side calories that usually accompany its consumption. We have also discussed how caffeine reduces your resting energy expenditure by breaking down muscle and by making muscle more difficult to build

167

and maintain. In the previous two chapters, we discussed the steps that we can take both to reduce our caffeine consumption, and to consume caffeine optimally, so that we can finally achieve a lean physique and keep it. By questioning and analyzing caffeine's impact on human energy balance, I think we have gained a better understanding of the causes and solutions to weight gain.

Some researchers believe that we are moving toward a new norm in which the average modern human is at least 50 pounds overweight, has type 2 diabetes, high blood pressure, joint problems, and a lower life expectancy.[222] It is striking that the epidemic of childhood obesity may help produce the first modern decline in American life expectancy. Let's avoid that future.

Misprints and Misconceptions

With regard to Mark Twain's statement about health books, I know that I am adding to an already large amount of information on this subject. Some of the information out there is misleading, to say the least. The notions that calories don't matter and that body composition is a frame of mind are good examples. As nice as it would be to think ourselves thin, that just isn't how it works.

Thinking is the first step to accomplishing most things in life, but thinking by itself is not enough without taking the appropriate actions. There are even some diet gurus who tell us that we are fat because we think that is what we deserve in life, or because we are afraid to be thin. Weight gain and weight loss are biological phenomena. If you read a book that tells you that "it's all in your head," you may get the misimpression that you can think yourself thin on the drive-thru diet.

So take in all the information you can and be discerning and careful. Keep that which works and discard that which does not. I hope that you keep at least some of the information in this book, and that it serves you well.

Take Care,

Eugene Wells

REFERENCES

1
Pendergrast, Mark. *Uncommon Grounds: The History of Coffee and How It Transformed Our World.* New York: Basic, 2000. 8. This was the Pope's supposed response to his priests who asked him to ban coffee.

2
Heymsfield, S., Darby, P., Muhlheim, L., et al. "The calorie: myth, measurement, and reality." *Am J Clin Nutr* 62 (1995): 1034S–41S.

3
Heymsfield, S., Darby, P., Muhlheim, L., et al. "The calorie: myth, measurement, and reality." *Am J Clin Nutr* 62 (1995): 1034S–41S.

Forbes, G. "Diet and exercise in obese subjects: self-report versus controlled measurements." *Nutr Rev* 51 (1993): 296-300.

Livingstone, M., Prentice, A., Strain, J., et al. "Accuracy of weighed dietary records in studies of diet and health." *Br Med J* 300 (1990): 708-12.

Bandini, L., Schoeller, D., Dyr, H., et al. "Validity of reported energy intake in obese and nonobese adolescents." *Am J Clin Nutr* 52 (1990): 421-5.

170

Black, A., Goldberg, O., Jebb, S., et al. "Critical evaluation of energy intake data using fundamental principles of energy physiology: 2. evaluating the results of published surveys." *Eur J Clin Nutr* 45 (1991): 583-99.

Lichtman, S., Pisarska, K., Berman, E., et al. "Discrepancy between self-reported and actual caloric intake and exercise in obese subjects." *N Engl J Med* 327 (1992): 1893-8.

Black, A., Prentice, A., Goldberg, O., et al. "Measurements of total energy expenditure provide insights into the validity of dietary measurements of energy intake." *J Am Diet Assoc* 93 (993): 572-9.

Goldberg, O., Black, A., Jebb, S., et al. "Critical evaluation of energy intake data using fundamental principles of energy physiology: 1. derivation of cut-off limits to identify under-recording." *Eur J Clin Nutr* 45 (1991): 569-81.

Lissner, L., Habicht, J., Strupp, B., et al. "Body composition and energy intake: do overweight women overeat and underreport?" *Am J Clin Nutr* 49 (1989): 320-5.

Livingstone, M., Prentice, A., Coward, W., et al. "Validation of estimates of energy intake by weighed dietary record and diet history in children and adolescents." *Am J Clin Nutr* 56 (1992): 29-35.

Schoeller, D. "How accurate is self-reported dietary energy intake?" *Nutr Rev* 48 (1990): 373-9.

Schoeller, D., Bandini, L., Dietz, W., et al. "Inaccuracies in self-reported intake identified by comparison with the doubly labelled water method." *Can J Physiol Pharmacol* 68 (1990): 941-9.

171

4

Heymsfield, S., Darby, P., Muhlheim, L., et al. "The calorie: myth, measurement, and reality." *Am J Clin Nutr* 62 (1995): 1034S–41S.

Rothblum, E. "Women and weight: fad and fiction." *J Psychol* 124 (1989): 5-24.

Shah, M., Jeffery, R. "Is obesity due to overeating and inactivity, or to a defective metabolic rate: a review." *Ann Behav Med* 13 (1991): 73-81.

Dattilo, A. "Dietary fat and its relationship to body weight." *Nutrition Today* 1992, January/February: 13-9.

5

Heymsfield, S., Darby, P., Muhlheim, L., et al. "The calorie: myth, measurement, and reality." *Am J Clin Nutr* 62 (1995): 1034S–41S.

6

Heymsfield, S., Darby, P., Muhlheim, L., et al. "The calorie: myth, measurement, and reality." *Am J Clin Nutr* 62 (1995): 1034S–41S.

Schoeller, D. "Limitations in the assessment of dietary energy intake by self-report." *Metabolism* 44 (1995): 18–22.

7

Buchholz, A., Schoeller, D. "Is a calorie a calorie?" *Am J Clin Nutr* 79 (2004): S899–906.

Kempen, K., Saris, W., Westerterp, K. "Energy balance during an 8-wk energy-restricted diet with and without exercise in obese women." *Am J Clin Nutr* 62 (1995): 722–9.

Heymsfield, S., Darby, P., Muhlheim, L., et al. "The calorie: myth, measurement, and reality." *Am J Clin Nutr* 62 (1995): 1034S–41S.

Clark, D., Tomas, F., Withers, R., et al. "Energy metabolism in free-living, 'large-eating' and 'small-eating' women: studies using $^2H_2(^{18})O$." *Br J Nutr* 72 (1994): 21–31.

Racette, S., Schoeller, D., Kushner, R., et al. "Exercise enhances dietary compliance during moderate energy restriction in obese women." *Am J Clin Nutr* 62 (1995): 345–9.

Mertz, W., Tsui, J., Judd, J., et al. "What are people really eating? The relation between energy intake derived from estimated diet records and intake determined to maintain body weight." *Am J Clin Nutr* 54 (1991): 291–5.

8
Heymsfield, S., Darby, P., Muhlheim, L., et al. "The calorie: myth, measurement, and reality." *Am J Clin Nutr* 62 (1995): 1034S–41S.

9
Ravussin, E., Lillioja, S., Anderson, T., et al. "Determinants of 24-hour energy expenditure in man: methods and results results using a respiratory chamber." *J Clin Invest* 78 (1986): 1568-78.

Forbes, G. "Diet and exercise in obese subjects: self-report versus controlled measurements." *Nutr Rev* 51 (1993): 296-300.

Lichtman, S., Pisarska, K., Berman, E., et al. "Discrepancy between self-reported and actual caloric intake and exercise in obese subjects." *N Engl J Med* 327 (1992): 1893-8.

173

Schoeller, D. "How accurate is self-reported dietary energy intake?" *Nutr Rev* 48 (1990): 373-9.

Schoeller, D., Bandini, L., Dietz ,W., et al. "Inaccuracies in self-reported intake identified by comparison with the doubly labelled water method." *Can J Physiol Pharmacol* 68 (1990): 941-9.

Prentice, A., Black, A., Coward, W., et al. "High levels of energy expenditure in obese women." *Br Med J* 292 (1986): 983-7.

Ravussin, E., Burnand, B., Schutz, Y., et al. "Twenty-four-hour energy expenditure and resting metabolic rate in obese, moderately obese, and control subjects." *Am J Clin Nutr* 35 (1982): 566-73.

Bandini, L., Schoeller, D., Dietz, W. "Energy expenditure in obese and nonobese adolescents." *Pediatr Res* 27 (1990): 198-202.

Welle, S., Forbes, G., Statt, M., et al. "Energy expenditure under free-living conditions in normal-weight and over-weight women." *Am J Clin Nutr* 55 (1992): 14-21.

Hibbert, J., Broemeling, L., Isenberg, J., et al. "Determinants of free-living energy expenditure in normal weight and obese women measured by doubly labeled water." *Obesity Res* 2 (1994): 44-53.

10
Mertz, W., Tsui, J., Judd, J., et al. "What are people really eating? The relation between energy intake derived from estimated diet records and intake determined to maintain body weight." *Am J Clin Nutr* 54 (1991): 291-5.

Black, A., Prentice, A., Goldberg, O., et al. "Mcasurements of total energy expenditure provide insights into the validity of dietary measurements of energy intake." *J Am Diet Assoc* 93 (993): 572-9.

11
Heymsfield, S., Darby, P., Muhlheim, L., et al. "The calorie: myth, measurement, and reality." *Am J Clin Nutr* 62 (1995): 1034S–41S.

Cameron. R., Evers, S. "Self-report issues in obesity and weight management: state of the art and future directions." *Behav Assessment* 12 (1990): 91-106.

Paulhaus, D. "Measurement and control of response bias." Robinson, J., Shafer, P., Wrightsman, I., eds. *Measures of personality and social psychological attitudes*. New York: Academic Press (1991): 17-59.

Paulhaus, D. "Two-component models of socially desirable responding." *J Pers Soc Psychol* 46 (1984): 598-609.

Paulhaus, D. "Self-deception and impression management in test responses." Angleitner, A., Wiggins, J., eds. *Personality assessment via questionnaire.* (1986): 143-65.

Lewis, M., Saarni, C. *Lying and deception in everyday life.* New York: Guilford Press, 1993.

12
Heymsfield, S., Darby, P., Muhlheim, L., et al. "The calorie: myth, measurement, and reality." *Am J Clin Nutr* 62 (1995): 1034S–41S.

Burros, M. "Eating well: some bagels are hefty in calories." *New York Times* 1994 July 6: 4(col 3).

Allison, D., Heshka, S., Sepulveda, D., et al. "Counting calories-caveat emptor." *JAMA* 270 (1993): 1454-6.

13
Schoeller, D. "The importance of clinical research: the role of thermogenesis in human obesity." *Am J Clin Nutr* 73 (2001): 511-516.

Weinsier, R., Nagy, T., Hunter, G., et al. "Do adaptive changes in metabolic rate favor weight regain in weight-reduced individuals? An examination of the set-point theory." *Am J Clin Nutr* 72 (2000): 1088-1094.

Newburgh, L., Johnston, M. "Endogenous obesity-a misconception." *Ann Intern Med* 3 (1938): 815-25.

Gullick, A. "A study of weight regulation in the adult human body during over nutrition." *Am J Physiol* 60 (1922): 371–95.

Heymsfield, S., Darby, P., Muhlheim, L., et al. "The calorie: myth, measurement, and reality." *Am J Clin Nutr* 62 (1995): 1034S–41S.

Skov, A., Toubro, S., Buemann, B., et al. "Normal levels of energy expenditure in patients with reported "low metabolism."" *Clin Physiol* 17 (1997): 279–85.

Lichtman, S., Pisarska, K., Berman, E., et al. "Discrepancy between self-reported and actual caloric intake and exercise in obese subjects." *N Engl J Med* 327 (1992): 1893-8.

Schoeller, D. "Measurement of energy expenditure in free-living humans by using doubly labeled water." *J Nutr* 118 (1988): 1278–89.

Coward, W., Roberts, S., Cole, T. "Theoretical and practical considerations in the doubly-labelled water ($^2H_2$ ^{18}O) method for the measurement of carbon dioxide production rate in man." *Eur J Clin Nutr* 42 (1987): 207–12.

Schoeller, D., van Santen, E. "Measurement of energy expenditure in humans by doubly labeled water method." *J Appl Physiol* 53 (1982): 955-9.

14

Ravussin, E., Schutz, Y., Acheson, K., et al. "Short-term, mixed-diet overfeeding in man: no evidence for "luxuskonsumption."" *Am J Physiol* 249 (1985): E470–7.

Schoeller, D. "The importance of clinical research: the role of thermogenesis in human obesity." *Am J Clin Nutr* 73 (2001): 511-516.

Schulz, L., Schoeller, D. "A compilation of total daily energy expenditures and body weights in healthy adults." *Am J Clin Nutr* 60 (1994): 676–81.

Prentice, A., Black, A., Coward, W., et al. "Energy expenditure in overweight and obese adults in affluent societies: an analysis of 319 doubly-labelled water measurements." *Eur J Clin Nutr* 50 (1996): 93–7.

Goran, M., Figueroa, R., McGloin, A., et al. "Obesity in children: recent advances in energy metabolism and body composition." *Obes Res* 3 (1995): 277-89.

Bandini, L., Schoeller, D., Edwards, J., et al. "Energy expenditure during carbohydrate overfeeding in obese and non-obese adolescents." *Am J Physiol* 256 (1989): E357–67.

Boutelle, K., Kirschenbaum, D. "Further support for consistent self-monitoring as a vital component of successful weight control." *Obes Res* 6 (1998): 219–224.

15
Weinsier, R., Nagy, T., Hunter, G., et al. "Do adaptive changes in metabolic rate favor weight regain in weight-reduced individuals? An examination of the set-point theory." *Am J Clin Nutr* 72 (2000): 1088-1094.

Wyatt, H., Grunwald, G., Seagle, H., et al. "Resting energy expenditure in reduced-obese subjects in the National Weight Control Registry." *Am J Clin Nutr* 69 (1999): 1189–93.

16
Ravussin, E., Schutz, Y., Acheson, K., et al. "Short-term, mixed-diet overfeeding in man: no evidence for "luxuskonsumption."" *Am J Physiol* 249 (1985): E470–7.

Ravussin, E., Lillioja, S., Anderson, T., et al. "Determinants of 24-hour energy expenditure in man: methods and results results using a respiratory chamber." *J Clin Invest* 78 (1986): 1568-78.

Saltzman, E., Roberts, S. "The role of energy expenditure in energy regulation: findings from a decade of research." *Nutr Rev* 53 (1995): 209–20.

17
Hill, J., Peters, J. "Environmental contributions to the obesity epidemic." *Science* 280 (1998): 1371–4.

Grundy, S. "Multifactorial causation of obesity: implications for prevention." *Am J Clin Nutr* 67 (1998): 563S–72S.

DiPietro, L. "Physical activity in the prevention of obesity: current evidence and research issues." *Med Sci Sports Exerc* 31 (1999): S542–6.

18
MacLean, P., Higgins, J., Wyatt, H., et al. "Regular exercise attenuates the metabolic drive to regain weight after long-term weight loss." *Am J Physiol Regul Integr Comp Physiol* 297 (2009): R793-R802.

19
Heymsfield, S., Darby, P., Muhlheim, L., et al. "The calorie: myth, measurement, and reality." *Am J Clin Nutr* 62 (1995): 1034S–41S.

Buhl, K., Gallagher, D., Matthews, D., et al. "Unexplained disturbance in body weight regulation: diagnostic outcome in patients referred for obesity evaluation reporting low energy intakes." *J Am Diet Assoc* (in press).

20
Westerterp, K., Wilson, S., Rolland, V. "Diet induced thermogenesis measured over 24 h in a respiration chamber: effect of diet composition." *Int J Obes* 23 (1999): 287-292.

Swaminathan, R., King, R., Holmfield, J., et al. "Thermic effect of feeding carbohydrate, fat, protein and mixed meal in lean and obese subjects." *Am J Clin Nutr* 42 (1985): 177–181.

Hill, J. "Understanding and Addressing the Epidemic of Obesity: An Energy Balance Perspective." *Endocrine Reviews* 27 (2006): 750-761.

Horton, T., Drougas, H., Brachey, A., et al. "Fat and carbohydrate overfeeding in humans: different effects on energy storage." *Am J Clin Nutr* 62 (1995): 19–29.

21

Heymsfield, S., Harp, J., Reitman, M., et al. "Why do obese patients not lose more weight when treated with low-calorie diets? A mechanistic perspective." *Am J Clin Nutr* 85 (2007): 346-354.

22

Bray, G. "Fructose: should we worry?" *Int J Obes.* 32 (2008): S127-31.

Levine, J. "Obesity: Mission Possible." *Diabetes* 56 (2007): 2653-2654.

23

Hill, J. "Understanding and Addressing the Epidemic of Obesity: An Energy Balance Perspective." *Endocrine Reviews* 27 (2006): 750-761.

24

Hill, J. "Understanding and Addressing the Epidemic of Obesity: An Energy Balance Perspective." *Endocrine Reviews* 27 (2006): 750-761.

Golay, A., Allaz, A., Morel, Y., et al. "Similar weight loss with low- or high-carbohydrate diets." *Am J Clin Nutr* 63 (1996): 174–178.

Kinsell, L., Gunning, B., Michaels, G., et al. "Calories do count." *Metabolism* 13 (1964): 195–204.

Garrow, J. *Treat obesity seriously: a clinical manual.* London: Churchill Livingstone, 1981.

25

Boden, G., Sargrad, K., Homko, C., et al. "Effect of a low-carbohydrate diet on appetite, blood glucose levels, and insulin resistance in obese patients with type 2 diabetes." *Ann Intern Med* 142 (2005): 403-11.

Buchholz, A., Schoeller, D. "Is a calorie a calorie?" *Am J Clin Nutr* 79 (2004): S899–906.

Schoeller, D., Buchholz, A.. "Energetics of obesity and weight control: does diet composition matter?" *J Am Diet Assoc* 105 (2005): S24–8.

Layman, D., Evans, E., Erickson, D., et al. "A Moderate-Protein Diet Produces Sustained Weight Loss and Long-Term Changes in Body Composition and Blood Lipids in Obese Adults." *Journal of Nutrition* 139 (2009): 514-521.

26
Aston, L., Stokes, C., Jebb, S. "No effect of a diet with a reduced glycaemic index on satiety, energy intake and body weight in overweight and obese women." *International Journal of Obesity* 32 (2008): 160-165.

Sloth, B., Krog-Mikkelsen, I., Flint, A., et al. "No difference in body weight decrease between a low-glycemic-index and a high-glycemic-index diet but reduced LDL cholesterol after 10-wk ad libitum intake of the low-glycemic-index diet." *Am J Clin Nutr* 80 (2004): 337-347.

Raben, A. "Should obese patients be counselled to follow a low-glycaemic index diet? No." *Obes Rev* 3 (2002): 245-56.

Raatz, S., Torkelson, C., Redmon, J., et al. "Reduced glycemic index and glycemic load diets do not increase the effects of energy restriction on weight loss and insulin sensitivity in obese men and women." *J Nutr* 135 (2005): 2387-91.

Ebbeling, C., Leidig, M., Feldman, H., et al. "Effects of a Low–Glycemic Load vs Low-Fat Diet in Obese Young Adults." *JAMA*. 297 (2007): 2092-2102.

27
Dansinger, M., Gleason, J., Griffith, J., et al. "Comparison of the Atkins, Ornish, Weight Watchers, and Zone diets for weight loss and heart disease risk reduction: a randomized trial." *JAMA* 293 (2005): 43–53.

28
Diaz, E., Galgani, J., Aguirre, C. "Glycaemic index effects on fuel partitioning in humans." *Obes Rev* 7 (2006): 219-26.

Galgani, J., Diaz, E., Aguirre, C. "Nutrition Discussion Forum." *British Journal of Nutrition* 95 (2006): 845–846.

29
Aston, L., Stokes, C., Jebb, S. "No effect of a diet with a reduced glycaemic index on satiety, energy intake and body weight in overweight and obese women." *International Journal of Obesity* 32 (2008): 160-165.

Sloth, B., Krog-Mikkelsen, I., Flint, A., et al. "No difference in body weight decrease between a low-glycemic-index and a high-glycemic-index diet but reduced LDL cholesterol after 10-wk ad libitum intake of the low-glycemic-index diet." *Am J Clin Nutr* 80 (2004): 337-347.

Raben, A. "Should obese patients be counselled to follow a low-glycaemic index diet? No." *Obes Rev* 3 (2002): 245-56.

Raatz, S., Torkelson, C., Redmon, J., et al. "Reduced glycemic index and glycemic load diets do not increase the effects of energy restriction on weight loss and insulin sensitivity in obese men and women." *J Nutr* 135 (2005): 2387-91.

Ebbeling, C., Leidig, M., Feldman, H., et al. "Effects of a Low–Glycemic Load vs Low-Fat Diet in Obese Young Adults." *JAMA*. 297 (2007): 2092-2102.

30
Hill, J., Wyatt, H." Outpatient management of obesity: a primary care perspective." *Obes Res* 10 (2002): 124S–30S.

Berkel, L., Poston, W., Reeves, R., et al. "Behavioral interventions for obesity." *J Am Diet Assoc* 105 (2005): S35–43.

Stunkard, A., McLaren-Hume, M. "The results of treatment for obesity." *Arch Intern Med* 103 (1959): 79–85.

Avenell, A., Broom, J., Brown, T., et al. "Systematic review of the long-term effects and economic consequences of treatments for obesity and implications for health improvement." *Health Technol Assess* 8 (2004): iii–iv, 1–182.

31
Heymsfield, S., Harp, J., Reitman, M., et al. "Why do obese patients not lose more weight when treated with low-calorie diets? A mechanistic perspective." *Am J Clin Nutr*. 85 (2007): 346-354.

Dansinger, M., Gleason, J., Griffith, J., et al. "Comparison of the Atkins, Ornish, Weight Watchers, and Zone diets for weight loss and heart disease risk reduction: a randomized trial." *JAMA* 293 (2005): 43–53.

32
Dansinger, M., Gleason, J., Griffith, J., et al. "Comparison of the Atkins, Ornish, Weight Watchers, and Zone diets for

weight loss and heart disease risk reduction: a randomized trial." *JAMA* 293 (2005): 43–53.

33
Foster, G., Wyatt, H., Hill, J., et al. "A multi-center, randomized, controlled clinical trial of the Atkin's diet." *N Engl J Med* 348 (2003): 282–290.

Stern, L., Iqbal, N., Seshadri, P., et al. "The effects of low carbohydrate versus conventional weight loss in severely obese adults: one year follow-up of a randomized trail." *Ann Intern Med* 140 (2004): 778–785.

Samaha, F., Iqbal, N., Seshadri, P., et al. "A low carbohydrate as compared to a low fat diet in severe obesity." *N Engl J Med* 348 (2003): 2074–2081.

Wing, R., Wadden, T. "Treatment of obesity by moderate and severe caloric restriction in weight loss and control: results of clinical research trials." *Ann Intern Med* 119 (1993): 688–693.

34
Foster, G., Wyatt, H., Hill, J., et al. "A multi-center, randomized, controlled clinical trial of the Atkin's diet." *N Engl J Med* 348 (2003): 282–290.

Stern, L., Iqbal, N., Seshadri, P., et al. "The effects of low carbohydrate versus conventional weight loss in severely obese adults: one year follow-up of a randomized trail." *Ann Intern Med* 140 (2004): 778–785.

Samaha, F., Iqbal, N., Seshadri, P., et al. "A low carbohydrate as compared to a low fat diet in severe obesity." *N Engl J Med* 348 (2003): 2074–2081.

35
Buchholz, A., Schoeller, D. "Is a calorie a calorie?" *Am J Clin Nutr* 79 (2004): S899–906.

Eisenstein, J., Roberts, S., Dallal, G., et al. "High-protein weight-loss diets: are they safe and do they work? A review of the experimental and epidemiologic data." *Nutr Rev* 60 (2002): 189–200.

Yao, M., Roberts, S. "Dietary energy density and weight regulation." *Nutr Rev* 59 (2001): 247–58.

Skov, A., Toubro, S., Ronn, B., et al. "Randomized trial on protein vs carbohydrate in ad libitum fat reduced diet for the treatment of obesity." *Int J Obes Relat Metab Disord* 23 (1999): 528–36.

Steiniger, J., Karst, H., Noack, R., et al. "Diet induced thermogenesis in man: thermic effects of single protein and carbohydrate test meals in lean and obese subjects." *Ann Nutr Metab* 31(1987): 117–125.

Schutz, Y., Bray, G., Margen, S. "Postprandial thermogenesis at rest and during exercise in elderly men ingesting two levels of protein." *J Am Col Nutr* 6 (1987): 497–506.

Robinson, S., Jaccard, C., Persaud, C., et al. "Protein turnover and thermogenesis in response to high protein and high carbohydrate feeding in man." *Am J Clin Nutr* 52 (1990): 72–80.

Halton, T., Hu, F. "The Effects of High Protein Diets on Thermogenesis, Satiety and Weight Loss: A Critical Review." *Journal of the American College of Nutrition* 23 (2004): 373-385.

185

Luscombe, N., Clifton, P., Noakes, M., et al: "Effect of a high protein, energy restricted diet on weight loss and energy expenditure after weight stabilization in hyperinsulinemic subjects." *Int J Obes* 27 (2003): 582–590.

Nair, K., Halliday, D., Garrow, J: "Thermic response to isoenergetic protein, carbohydrate or fat meals in lean and obese subjects." *Clin Sci* 65 (1983): 307–312.

Westerterp, K., Wilson, S., Rolland, V. "Diet induced thermogenesis measured over 24 h in a respiration chamber: effect of diet composition." *Int J Obes* 23 (1999): 287-292.

Crovetti, R., Porrini, M., Santangelo, A., et al. "The influence of thermic effect of food on satiety." *Euro J Clin Nutr* 52 (1997): 482–488.

Daucey, M., Bingham, S. "Dependence of 24 h energy expenditure in man on the composition of the nutrient intake." *Br J Nutr* 50 (1983): 1–13.

Karst, H., Steiniger, J., Noack, R., et al. "Diet induced thermogenesis in man: thermic effects of single proteins, carbohydrates and fats depending on their energy amount." *Ann Nutr Metab* 28 (1984): 245–252.

Weigle, D., Breen, P., Matthys, C., et al. "A high-protein diet induces sustained reductions in appetite, ad libitum caloric intake, and body weight despite compensatory changes in diurnal plasma leptin and ghrelin concentrations." *Am J Clin Nutr* 82 (2005): 41–8.

Adam-Perrot, A., Clifton, P., Brouns, F. "Low-carbohydrate diets: nutritional and physiological aspects." *Obes Rev* 7 (2006): 49–58.

36
Westerterp-Plantenga, M., Rolland, V., Wilson, S., et al. "Satiety related to 24-h diet-induced thermogenesis during high protein/carbohydrate vs high fat diets measured in a respiratory chamber." *Eur J Clin Nutr* 53 (1999): 495–502.

Mikkelsen, P., Toubro, S., Astrup, A. "The effect of fat-reduced diets on 24-h energy expenditure: comparisons between animal protein, vegetable protein, and carbohydrate." *Am J Clin Nutr* 72 (2000):1135–41.

Feinman, R., Fine, E. "Thermodynamics and metabolic advantage of weight loss diets." *Metab Syndr Relat Disord* 1 (2003): 209–19.

Whitehead, J., McNeill, G., Smith, J. "The effect of protein intake on 24-h energy expenditure during energy restriction." *Int J Obes Relat Metab Disord* 20 (1996): 727–32.

Eisenstein, J., Roberts, S., Dallal, G., et al. "High-protein weight-loss diets: are they safe and do they work? A review of the experimental and epidemiologic data." *Nutr Rev* 60 (2002): 189–200.

37
Layman, D., Boileau, R., Erickson, D., et al. "A reduced ratio of dietary carbohydrate to protein improves body composition and blood lipid profiles during weight loss in adult women." *J Nutr* 133 (2003): 411–7.

Layman, D., Evans, E., Baum, J., et al. "Dietary protein and exercise have additive effects on body composition during weight loss in adult women." *J Nutr* 135 (2005): 1903–10.

Westerterp-Plantenga, M., Lejeune, M., Nigs, I., et al. "High protein intake sustains weight maintenance after body weight loss in humans." *Int J Obes Relat Metab Disord* 28 (2004): 57–64.

Millward, D. "An adaptive metabolic demand model for protein and amino acid requirements." *Br J Nutr* 90 (2003): 249–60.

Layman, D. "Protein quantity and quality at levels above the RDA improves adult weight loss." *J Am Coll Nutr* 23 (2004): S631–6.

38
Buchholz, A., Schoeller, D. "Is a calorie a calorie?" *Am J Clin Nutr* 79 (2004): S899–906.

Davy, K., Horton, T., Davy, B., et al. "Regulation of macronutrient balance in healthy young and older men." *Int J Obes Relat Metab Disord* 25 (2001): 1497–502.

Roy, H., Lovejoy, J., Keenan, M., et al. "Substrate oxidation and energy expenditure in athletes and nonathletes consuming isoenergetic high- and low-fat diets." *Am J Clin Nutr* 67 (1998): 405–11.

Thomas, C., Peters, J., Reed, G., et al. "Nutrient balance and energy expenditure during ad libitum feeding of high-fat and high-carbohydrate diets in humans." *Am J Clin Nutr* 55 (1992): 934–42.

Hill, J., Peters, J., Reed, G., et al. "Nutrient balance in humans: effects of diet composition." *Am J Clin Nutr* 54 (1991): 10–17.

Rumpler, W., Seale, J., Miles, C., et al. "Energy-intake restriction and diet-composition effects on energy expenditure in men." *Am J Clin Nutr* 53 (1991): 430–6.

Lean, M., James, W. "Metabolic effects of isoenergetic nutrient exchange over 24 hours in relation to obesity in women." *Int J Obes* 12 (1988): 15–27.

Abbott, W., Howard, B., Ruotolo, G., et al. "Energy expenditure in humans: effects of dietary fat and carbohydrate." *Am J Physiol* 258 (1990): E347–51.

Verboeket-van de Venne, W., Westerterp, K. "Effects of dietary fat and carbohydrate exchange on human energy metabolism." *Appetite* 26 (1996): 287–300.

Astrup, A., Buemann, B., Christensen, N., et al. "Failure to increase lipid oxidation in response to increasing dietary fat content in formerly obese women." *Am J Physiol* 266 (1994): E592–9.

Whitehead, J., McNeill, G., Smith, J. "The effect of protein intake on 24-h energy expenditure during energy restriction." *Int J Obes Relat Metab Disord* 20 (1996): 727–32.

39
Buchholz, A., Schoeller, D. "Is a calorie a calorie?" *Am J Clin Nutr* 79 (2004): S899–906.

40
Haugen, H., Melanson, E., Tran, Z. "Variability of measured resting metabolic rate." *Am J Clin Nutr* 78 (2003): 1141-1145.

41
Hill, J. "Understanding and Addressing the Epidemic of Obesity: An Energy Balance Perspective." *Endocrine Reviews* 27 (2006): 750-761.

Di Pietro, L., Dziura, J., Blair, S. "Estimated change in physical activity levels (PAL) and prediction of 5-year weight change in men: the aerobics center longitudinal study." *Int J Obes Relat Metab Disord* 28 (2004): 1541–1547.

French, S., Jeffery, R., Forster, J., et al. "Predictors of weight change over two years among a population of working adults: the Healthy Worker Project." *Int J Obes Relat Metab Disord* 18 (1994): 145–154.

Hill, J., Wyatt, H. "Role of physical activity in preventing and treating obesity." *J Appl Phyisol* 99 (2005): 765–770.

Horton, T., Hill, J. "Exercise and obesity." *Proc Nutr Soc* 57 (1998): 85–91.

Hill, J., Davis, J., Tagliaferro, A. "Effects of diet and exercise training on thermogenesis in adult female rats." *Physiol Behav* 31 (1983): 133–135.

Murgatroyd, P., Goldberg, G., Leahy, F., et al. "Effects of inactivity and diet composition on human energy balance." *Int J Obes Relat Metab Disord* 23 (1999): 1269–1275.

42
Smith, Barry D., Tola, Kenneth. "Caffeine: Effects on Psychological Functioning and Performance." *Caffeine*. Ed. Gene A. Spiller. Florida: CRC Press, 1998.

43
Weinberg, Bennett Alan, Bealer, Bonnie K. *The World of Caffeine: The Science and Culture of the World's Most Popular Drug*. New York: Routledge, 2001. 235.

44
Weinberg and Bealer, xiii-xix.

45
Tarka, Stanley M., Hurst, W. Jeffrey. "Introduction to the Chemistry, Isolation, and Biosynthesis of Methylxanthines." *Caffeine*. Ed. Gene A. Spiller. Florida: CRC Press, 1998.

46
Lundsberg, Lisbet S. "Caffeine Consumption." *Caffeine*. Ed. Gene A. Spiller. Florida: CRC Press, 1998.

47
Weinberg and Bealer, 31.

48
Weinberg and Bealer, xii.

49
Lundsberg, Lisbet S. "Caffeine Consumption." *Caffeine*. Ed. Gene A. Spiller. Florida: CRC Press, 1998.

50
Weinberg and Bealer, xii.

51
Lundsberg, Lisbet S. "Caffeine Consumption." *Caffeine*. Ed. Gene A. Spiller. Florida: CRC Press, 1998.

Smith, Barry D., Tola, Kenneth. "Caffeine: Effects on Psychological Functioning and Performance." *Caffeine*. Ed. Gene A. Spiller. Florida: CRC Press, 1998.

52
Weinberg and Bealer, 28.

Lundsberg, Lisbet S. "Caffeine Consumption." *Caffeine*. Ed. Gene A. Spiller. Florida: CRC Press, 1998.

53
Hoffman, David Lee, "Tea in China." *Caffeine*. Ed. Gene A. Spiller. Florida: CRC Press, 1998.

54
Balentine, Douglas A., Harbowy, Matthew E., Graham, Harold N. "Tea: The Plant and its Manufacture; Chemistry and Consumption of the Beverage." *Caffeine*. Ed. Gene A. Spiller. Florida: CRC Press, 1998.

55
Weinberg and Bealer, xv.

Smit, H., Blackburn, R. "Reinforcing effects of caffeine and theobromine as found in chocolate." *Psychopharmacology* (Berl) 181 (2005): 101-6.

56
Apgar, Joan L., Tarka, Stanley M. "Methylxanthine Composition and Consumption Patterns of Cocoa and Chocolate Products." *Caffeine*. Ed. Gene A. Spiller. Florida: CRC Press, 1998.

57
Weinberg and Bealer, 55.

58
Apgar, Joan L., Tarka, Stanley M. "Methylxanthine Composition and Consumption Patterns of Cocoa and Chocolate Products." *Caffeine*. Ed. Gene A. Spiller. Florida: CRC Press, 1998.

59
Weinberg and Bealer, 3.

60
Smith, Barry D., Tola, Kenneth. "Caffeine: Effects on Psychological Functioning and Performance." *Caffeine*. Ed. Gene A. Spiller. Florida: CRC Press, 1998.
(Quoting Abd-al-Kadir, *In Praise of Coffee*, 1587.)

61
Smith, Barry D., Tola, Kenneth. "Caffeine: Effects on Psychological Functioning and Performance." *Caffeine*. Ed. Gene A. Spiller. Florida: CRC Press, 1998.

62
Lundsberg, Lisbet S. "Caffeine Consumption." *Caffeine*. Ed. Gene A. Spiller. Florida: CRC Press, 1998.

63
Pendergrast, 15.

64
Weinberg and Bealer, 186-187.

65
Weinberg and Bealer, xiii.

66
Weinberg and Bealer, 190-191.

67
Pendergrast, 157.

68
Lundsberg, Lisbet S. "Caffeine Consumption." *Caffeine*. Ed. Gene A. Spiller. Florida: CRC Press, 1998.

69
Pendergrast, 420.

70
Weinberg and Bealer, 260.

71
Weinberg and Bealer, 198.

72
Apgar, Joan L., Tarka, Stanley M. "Methylxanthine Composition and Consumption Patterns of Cocoa and Chocolate Products." *Caffeine*. Ed. Gene A. Spiller. Florida: CRC Press, 1998.

Lundsberg, Lisbet S. "Caffeine Consumption." *Caffeine*. Ed. Gene A. Spiller. Florida: CRC Press, 1998.

73
Biaggioni, I., Davis, S. "Caffeine: A Cause of Insulin Resistance?" *Diabetes Care* 25 (2002): 399-40.

74
Apgar, Joan L., Tarka, Stanley M. "Methylxanthine Composition and Consumption Patterns of Cocoa and Chocolate Products." *Caffeine*. Ed. Gene A. Spiller. Florida: CRC Press, 1998.

75
Lundsberg, Lisbet S. "Caffeine Consumption." *Caffeine*. Ed. Gene A. Spiller. Florida: CRC Press, 1998.

76
Weinberg and Bealer, 203.

77
Weinberg and Bealer, 198.

78
Weinberg and Bealer, xiii.

Smith, Barry D., Tola, Kenneth. "Caffeine: Effects on Psychological Functioning and Performance." *Caffeine.* Ed. Gene A. Spiller. Florida: CRC Press, 1998.

79
Smith, Barry D., Tola, Kenneth. "Caffeine: Effects on Psychological Functioning and Performance." *Caffeine.* Ed. Gene A. Spiller. Florida: CRC Press, 1998.

80
Smith, Barry D., Tola, Kenneth. "Caffeine: Effects on Psychological Functioning and Performance." *Caffeine.* Ed. Gene A. Spiller. Florida: CRC Press, 1998.

81
Stephen Cherniske. *Caffeine Blues: Wake Up to the Hidden Dangers of America's #1 Drug.* New York: Warner Books, 1998. 51.

Vincent-Viry, M., Pontes, Z., Gueguen, R., et al. "Segregation analyses of four urinary caffeine metabolite ratios implicated in the determination of human acetylation phenotypes." *Genet Epidemiol* 11 (1994): 115-29.

82
Hildebrand, M., Seifert, W. "Determination of acetylator phenotype in Caucasians with caffeine." *European Journal of Clinical Pharmacology* 37 (1989): 525-526.

See also Rieder, M., Shear, N., Kanee, A. et al. "Prominence of slow acetylator phenotype among patients with sulfonamide hypersensitivity reactions." *Clin Pharmacol Ther* 49 (1991): 13-7.

83
Smith, Barry D., Tola, Kenneth. "Caffeine: Effects on Psychological Functioning and Performance." *Caffeine*. Ed. Gene A. Spiller. Florida: CRC Press, 1998.

84
Smith, Barry D., Tola, Kenneth. "Caffeine: Effects on Psychological Functioning and Performance." *Caffeine*. Ed. Gene A. Spiller. Florida: CRC Press, 1998.

85
Spiller, Gene A. "Basic Metabolism and Physiological Effects of the Methylxanthines." *Caffeine*. Ed. Gene A. Spiller. Florida: CRC Press, 1998.

"Caffeine Can Increase Brain Serotonin Levels." *Nutrition Reviews* 46 (1988): 366-67.

86
Weinberg and Bealer, 235.

87
Weinberg and Bealer, 237.

88
Weinberg and Bealer, 237.

89
Lundsberg, Lisbet S. "Caffeine Consumption." *Caffeine*. Ed. Gene A. Spiller. Florida: CRC Press, 1998.

90
Spiller, Gene A. "Caffeine Content of some Cola Beverages." *Caffeine*. Ed. Gene A. Spiller. Florida: CRC Press, 1998.

91
Lundsberg, Lisbet S. "Caffeine Consumption." *Caffeine.* Ed. Gene A. Spiller. Florida: CRC Press, 1998.

92
Maglione-Garves, C., Kravitz, L., Schneider, S. "Cortisol Connection: Tips on Managing Stress and Weight." *The University of New Mexico: Selected Articles by Len Kravitz and Colleagues.* Ed. Len Kravitz. August 1, 2010. <http://www.unm.edu/~lkravitz/Article%20folder/stresscortisol.html>.

93
Lovallo, W., Whitsett, T., al'Absi, M., et al. "Caffeine Stimulation of Cortisol Secretion Across the Waking Hours in Relation to Caffeine Intake Levels." *Psychosom Med* 67 (2005): 734-9.

Talbott, Shawn. *The Cortisol Connection: Why Stress Makes You Fat and Ruins Your Health – and What You Can Do About It.* Alameda: Hunter House, 2002. 28.

Henry, J., Stephens, P: "Caffeine as an intensifier of stress-induced hormonal and pathopysiologic changes in mice." *Pharmacol Biochem Behav* 13 (1980): 719-727.

Slivka, D., Hailes, W., Cuddy, J., et al. "Caffeine and carbohydrate supplementation during exercise when in negative energy balance: effects on performance, metabolism, and salivary cortisol." *Appl Physiol Nutr Metab* 33 (2008): 079-85.

Beaven, C., Hopkins, W., Hansen, K., et al. "Dose effect of caffeine on testosterone and cortisol responses to resistance exercise." *Int J Sport Nutr Exerc Metab* 18 (2008): 131-41.

197

Lane, J., Adcock, R., Williams, R., et al. "Caffeine effects on cardiovascular and neuroendocrine responses to acute psychosocial stress and their relationship to level of habitual caffeine consumption." *Psychosomatic Medicine* 52 (1990): 320-336.

al'Absi, M., Lovallo, W., McKey, B., et al. "Hypothalamic-pituitary-adrenocortical responses to psychological stress and caffeine in men at high and low risk for hypertension." *Psychosomatic Medicine* 60 (1998): 521-527.

al'Absi, M., Lovallo, W., Pincomb, G., et al. "Adrenocortical effects of caffeine at rest and during mental stress in borderline hypertensive men." *Int J Behav Med* 2 (1995): 263-275.

Lovallo, W., al'Absi, M., Blick, K., et al. "Stress-like adrenocorticotropin responses to caffeine in young healthy men." *Pharmacol Biochem Behav* 55 (1996): 365-9.

Lovallo, W., Pincomb, G., Sung, B., et al. "Caffeine may potentiate adrenocortical stress responses in hypertension-prone men." *Hypertension* 14 (1989): 170-6.

Pincomb, G., Lovallo, W., Passey, R., et al. "Caffeine enhances the physiological response to occupational stress in medical students." *Health Psychol* 6 (1987): 101-12.

Shepard, J., al'Absi, M., Whitsett, T., et al. "Additive pressor effects of caffeine and stress in male medical students at risk for hypertension." *Am J Hypertens* 13 (2000): 475-81.

Lucas, P., Pickar, D., Kelsoe, J., et al. "Effects of the acute administration of caffeine in patients with schizophrenia." *Biol Psychiatry* 28 (1990): 35-40.

94
Lovallo, W., al'Absi, M., Blick, K., et al. "Stress-like adreno-corticotropin responses to caffeine in young healthy men." *Pharmacol Biochem Behav* 55 (1996): 365-9.

Talbott, 104.

95
Anagnostis, P., Athyros, V., Tziomalos, K., et al. "Clinical review: The pathogenetic role of cortisol in the metabolic syndrome: a hypothesis." *J Clin Endocrinol Metab* 94 (2009): 2692-701.

Walker, B. "Cortisol--cause and cure for metabolic syndrome?" *Diabet Med* 23 (2006): 1281-8.

De Vriendt, T., Moreno, L., De Henauw, S. "Chronic stress and obesity in adolescents: scientific evidence and methodological issues for epidemiological research." *Nutr Metab Cardiovasc Dis* 19 (2009): 511-9.

Talbott, 28.

Björntorp, P. "Do stress reactions cause abdominal obesity and comorbidities?" *Obes Rev* 2 (2001): 73-86.

Ljung, T., Ottosson, M., Ahlberg, A., et al. "Central and peripheral glucocorticoid receptor function in abdominal obesity." *J Endocrinol Invest* 25 (2002): 229-35.

Björntorp, P., Rosmond, R. "The metabolic syndrome--a neuroendocrine disorder?" *Br J Nutr* 83 (2000): S49-57.

Vgontzas, A., Bixler, E. "Short Sleep and Obesity: Are Poor Sleep, Chronic Stress, and Unhealthy Behaviors the Link?" *Sleep* 31 (2008): 1203.

96
Cherniske, 226.

97
Talbott, 86.

98
Björntorp, P., Rössner, S., Uddén, J. ["Consolatory eating" is not a myth. Stress-induced increased cortisol levels result in leptin-resistant obesity] *Lakartidningen* 98 (2001): 5458-61.

Leal-Cerro, A., Soto, A., Martínez, M., et al. "Influence of Cortisol Status on Leptin Secretion." *Pituitary* 4 (2001): 111-116.

99
MacLean, P., Higgins, J., Johnson, G., et al. "Enhanced metabolic efficiency contributes to weight regain after weight loss in obesity-prone rats." *Am J Physiol* 287 (2004): R1306–R1315.

MacLean, P., Higgins, J., Johnson, G., et al. "Metabolic adjustments with the development, treatment, and recurrence of obesity in obesity-prone rats." *Am J Physiol* 287 (2004): R288–R297.

MacLean, P., Higgins, J., Jackman, M., et al. "Peripheral metabolic responses to prolonged weight reduction that promote rapid, efficient regain in obesity-prone rats." *Am J Physiol* 290 (2006): R1577–R1588.

100
Talbott, 29, 190.

Epel, E., Lapidus, R., McEwen, B., et al. "Stress may add bite to appetite in women: a laboratory study of stress-induced cortisol and eating behavior." *Psychoneuroendocrinology* 26 (2001): 37-49.

Newman, E., O'Connor, D., Conner, M. "Daily hassles and eating behaviour: the role of cortisol reactivity status." *Psychoneuroendocrinology* 32 (2007): 125-32.

Gluck, M. "Stress response and binge eating disorder." *Appetite* 46 (2006): 26-30.

Gluck, M., Geliebter, A., Hung, J., et al. "Cortisol, hunger, and desire to binge eat following a cold stress test in obese women with binge eating disorder." *Psychosom Med* 66 (2004): 876-81.

Dallman, M., la Fleur, S., Pecoraro, N., et al. "Minireview: Glucocorticoids—food intake, abdominal obesity, and wealthy nations in 2004." *Endocrinology* 145 (2004): 2633–2638.

Levine, M., Marcus, M. "Eating behavior following stress in women with and without bulimic symptoms." *Ann Behav Med* 19 (1997): 132–8.

Tataranni, P., Larson, D., Snitker, S., et al. "Effects of glucocorticoids on energy metabolism and food intake in humans." *Am J Physiol* 271 (1996): E317–25.

Cattanach, L., Malley, R., Rodin, J. "Psychologic and physiologic reactivity to stressors in eating disordered individuals." *Psychosom Med* 50 (1988): 591–9.

Lingswiler, V., Crowther, J., Stephens, M. "Emotional reactivity and eating in binge eating and obesity." *J Behav Med* 10 (1987): 287–99.

Telch, C., Agras, W. "Do emotional states influence binge eating in the obese?" *Int J Eat Disord* 20 (1996): 271–9.

Pirke, K., Platte, P., Laessle, R., et al. "The effect of a mental challenge test of plasma norepinephrine and cortisol in bulimia nervosa and in controls." *Biol Psychiatry* 32 (1992): 202–6.

101
Talbott, 39.

Sved, F., Shawar, A. "The Acute Effect of a Noontime Meal on the Serum Levels of Cortisol and DHEA in Lean and Obese Women." *Psychoneuroendocrinolgy* 22 (1997): S115-119.

Ljung, T., Andersson, B., Bengtsson, B., et al. "Inhibition of cortisol secretion by dexamethasone in relation to body fat distribution: a dose-response study." *Obes Res* 4 (1996): 277-82.

102
Sen, Y., Aygun, D., Yilmaz, E., et al. "Children and adolescents with obesity and the metabolic syndrome have high circulating cortisol levels." *Neuro Endocrinol Lett* 29 (2008): 141-5.

See also Andrew, R., Phillips, D., Walker, B. "Obesity and gender influence cortisol secretion and metabolism in man." *J Clin Endocrinol Metab* 83 (1998): 1806-9.

103
Gluck, M., Geliebter, A., Lorence, M. "Cortisol stress response is positively correlated with central obesity in obese women with binge eating disorder (BED) before and after cognitive-behavioral treatment." *Ann N Y Acad Sci* 1032 (2004): 202-7.

104
Talbott, 33.

Ottosson, M., Lönnroth, P., Björntorp, P., et al. "Effects of cortisol and growth hormone on lipolysis in human adipose tissue." *J Clin Endocrinol Metab* 85 (2000): 799-803.

105
Talbott, 16, 36, 104.

Rosmond, R., Dallman, M., Björntorp, P. "Stress-related cortisol secretion in men: relationships with abdominal obesity and endocrine, metabolic and hemodynamic abnormalities." *J Clin Endocrinol Metab* 83 (1998): 1853-9.

Beaven, C., Hopkins, W., Hansen, K., et al. "Dose effect of caffeine on testosterone and cortisol responses to resistance exercise." *Int J Sport Nutr Exerc Metab* 18 (2008):131-41.

106
Talbott, 177.

107
Brillon, D., Zheng, B., Campbell, R., et al. "Effect of cortisol on energy expenditure and amino acid metabolism in humans." *Am J Physiol* 268 (1995): E501-13.

Simmons, P., Miles, J., Gerich, J., et al. "Increased proteolysis: an effect of increases in plasma cortisol within the physiological range." *J Clin Invest* 73 (1984): 412-420.

Jalali, Rehan. "Muscle Breakdown: Is Cortisol Leading You Down the Catabolic Pathway?" *MesoRx*. August 1, 2010. <http://www.mesomorphosis.com/articles/jalali/cortisol.htm>.

108
Maglione-Garves, C., Kravitz, L., Schneider, S. "Cortisol Connection: Tips on Managing Stress and Weight." *The University of New Mexico: Selected Articles by Len Kravitz and Colleagues*. Ed. Len Kravitz. August 1, 2010. <http://www.unm.edu/~lkravitz/Article%20folder/stresscortisol.html>.

109
Brillon, D., Zheng, B., Campbell, R., et al. "Effect of cortisol on energy expenditure and amino acid metabolism in humans." *Am J Physiol* 268 (1995): E501-13.

110
Simmons, P., Miles, J., Gerich, J., et al. "Increased proteolysis: an effect of increases in plasma cortisol within the physiological range." *J Clin Invest* 73 (1984): 412-420.

111
Weinberg and Bealer, 196.

112
Talbott, 39.

Swaab, D, Raadsheer, F., Endert, E., et al. "Increased Cortisol Levels in Aging and Alzheimer's Disease in Postmortem Cerebrospinal Fluid." *Journal of Neuroendocrinology* 6 (1994): 681-687.

113
Talbott, 41.

114
Epel, E., McEwen, B., Seeman, T., et al. "Stress and body shape: stress-induced cortisol secretion is consistently greater among women with central fat." *Psychosomatic Medicine* 62 (2000): 623-632.

Mayo-Smith, W., Hayes, C., Biller, B., et al. "Body fat distribution measured with CT: correlations in healthy subjects, patients with anorexia nervosa, and patients with Cushing syndrome." *Radiology* 170 (1989): 515–8.

Rebuffe-Scrive, M., Krotkiewski, M., Elfverson, J., et al. "Muscle and adipose tissue morphology and metabolism in Cushing's syndrome." *J Clin Endocrinol Metab* 67 (1988): 1122–8.

Thakore, J., Richards, P., Reznek, R., et al. "Increased intraabdominal fat in major depression." *Biol Psychiatry* 41 (1997): 1140–2.

Marin, P., Darin, N., Amemiya, T., et al. "Cortisol secretion in relation to body fat distribution in obese premenopausal women." *Metabolism* 41 (1992): 882–6.

Moyer, A., Rodin, J., Grilo, C., et al. "Stress-induced cortisol response and fat distribution in women." *Obes Res* 2 (1994): 255–62.

Szostak-Wegierek, D., Bjorntorp, P., Marin, P., et al. "Influence of smoking on hormone secretion in obese and lean female smokers." *Obes Res* 4 (1996): 321–8.

Ljung, T., Andersson, B., Bengtsson, B., et al. "Inhibition of cortisol secretion by dexamethasone in relation to body fat distribution: a dose-response study." *Obes Res* 4 (1996): 277–81.

Pasquali, R., Cantobelli, S., Casimirri, F., et al. "The hypothalamic-pituitary-adrenal axis in obese women with different patterns of body fat distribution." *J Clin Endocrinol Metab* 77 (1993): 341–6.

205

Rosmond, R., Björntorp, P. "Occupational status, cortisol secretory pattern, and visceral obesity in middle-aged men." *Obes Res.* 8 (2000): 445-50.

Davis, M., Twamley, E., Hamilton, N., et al. "Body fat distribution and hemodynamic stress responses in premenopausal obese women: a preliminary study." *Health Psychol* 18 (1999): 625–33.

Waldstein, S., Burns, H., Toth, M., et al. "Cardiovascular reactivity and central adiposity in older African Americans." *Health Psychol* 18 (1999): 221–8.

Jayo, J., Shively, C., Kaplan, J., et al. "Effects of exercise and stress on body fat distribution in male cynomolgus monkeys." *Int J Obes Relat Metab Disord* 17 (1993): 597–604.

Rebuffe-Scrive, M., Krotkiewski, M., Elfverson, J., et al. "Muscle and adipose tissue morphology and metabolism in Cushing's syndrome." *J Clin Endocrinol Metab* 67 (1988): 1122–8.

Rebuffe-Scrive, M., Walsh, U., McEwen, B., et al. "Effect of chronic stress and exogenous glucocorticoids on regional fat distribution and metabolism." *Physiol Behav* 52 (1992): 583–90.

Weber-Hamann, B., Hentschel, F., Kniest, A., et al. "Hypercortisolemic depression is associated with increased intra-abdominal fat." *Psychosom Med* 64 (2002): 274–7.

Wajchenberg, L. "Subcutaneous and visceral adipose tissue. Their relation to the metabolic syndrome." *Endocr Rev* 21 (2000): 697–738.

Rebuffé-Scrive, M., Bronnegard, M., Nilsson, A., et al. "Steroid hormone receptors in human adipose tissue." *J Clin Endocrinol Metab* 71 (1990): 1215–9.

Talbott, 39.

Geer, E., Shen, W., Gallagher, D., et al. "MRI Assessment of Lean and Adipose Tissue Distribution in Female Patients with Cushing's Disease." *Clin Endocrinol* 2010 Jun 9. (Ahead of print)

Anagnostis, P., Athyros, V., Tziomalos, K., et al. "Clinical review: The pathogenetic role of cortisol in the metabolic syndrome: a hypothesis." *J Clin Endocrinol Metab* 94 (2009): 2692-701.

De Vriendt, T., Moreno, L., De Henauw, S. "Chronic stress and obesity in adolescents: scientific evidence and methodological issues for epidemiological research." *Nutr Metab Cardiovasc Dis* 19 (2009): 511-9.

Jayo, J., Shively, C., Kaplan, J., et al. "Effects of exercise and stress on body fat distribution in male cynomolgus monkeys." *Int J Obes Relat Metab Disord* 17 (1993): 597–604.

Bjorntorp, P., Rosmond, R. "Neuroendocrine abnormalities in visceral obesity." *Int J Obes Relat Metab Disord* 24 (2000): S80–5.

Bjorntorp P. "Abdominal fat distribution and disease: an overview of epidemiological data." *Ann Med* 24 (1992): 15–8.

Wallerius, S., Rosmond, R., Ljung, T., et al. "Rise in morning saliva cortisol is associated with abdominal obesity in men: a preliminary report." *J Endocrinol Invest* 26 (2003): 616–9.

115
Epel, E., McEwen, B., Seeman, T., et al. "Stress and body shape: stress-induced cortisol secretion is consistently greater among women with central fat." *Psychosomatic Medicine* 62 (2000): 623-632.

Larsson, B., Svardsudd, L., Welin, L., et al. "Abdominal adipose tissue distribution, obesity, and risk of cardiovascular disease and death: a 13-year follow-up of participants in the study of men born in 1913." *BMJ* 288 (1984): 1401–4.

116
Jalali, Rehan. "Muscle Breakdown: Is Cortisol Leading You Down the Catabolic Pathway?" *MesoRx*. August 1, 2010. <http://www.mesomorphosis.com/articles/jalali/cortisol.htm>.

117
Talbott, 115, 118-119.

Carrillo, A., Murphy, R., Cheung, S. "Vitamin C supplementation and salivary immune function following exercise-heat stress." *Int J Sports Physiol Perform* 3 (2008): 516-30.

Cascalheira, J., Parreira, M., Viegas, A. et al. "Serum homocysteine: relationship with circulating levels of cortisol and ascorbate." *Ann Nutr Metab* 53 (2008): 67-74.

Nakhostin-Roohi, B., Babaei, P., Rahmani-Nia, F., et al. "Effect of vitamin C supplementation on lipid peroxidation, muscle damage and inflammation after 30-min exercise at

75% VO2max." *J Sports Med Phys Fitness* 48 (2008): 217-24.

118
Smith, Barry D., Tola, Kenneth. "Caffeine: Effects on Psychological Functioning and Performance." *Caffeine*. Ed. Gene A. Spiller. Florida: CRC Press, 1998.

119
Smith, Barry D., Tola, Kenneth. "Caffeine: Effects on Psychological Functioning and Performance." *Caffeine*. Ed. Gene A. Spiller. Florida: CRC Press, 1998.

120
Iancu, I., Dolberg, O., Zohar, J. "Is caffeine involved in the pathogenesis of combat-stress reaction?" *Mil Med* 161 (1996): 230-32.

121
Lane, J., Adcock, R., Williams, R., et al. "Caffeine effects on cardiovascular and neuroendocrine responses to acute psychosocial stress and their relationship to level of habitual caffeine consumption." *Psychosomatic Medicine* 52 (1990): 320-336.

122
Talbott, 30.

Cherniske, 59.

123
Talbott, 18.

Cherniske, 21.

124
Überт, S., Fuhlenriede, M., Becker, A., et al. "Is there an

inhibitory role of cortisol in the mechanism of male sexual arousal and penile erection?" *Urological Research* 31 (2003): 402-406.

Sapolsky, R. "Stress-induced suppression of testicular function in the wild baboon: role of glucocorticoids." *Endocrinology* 116 (1985): 2273–2278.

MacAdams, M., White, R., Chipps, B. "Reduction of serum testosterone levels during chronic glucocorticoid therapy." *Ann Intern Med* 104 (1986): 648–651.

Fitzgerald, R., Skingle, S., Crisp, A. "Testosterone concentrations in men on chronic glucocorticosteroid therapy." *J Royal Coll Physicians Lond* 31 (1997): 168–170.

Lac, G., Berthon, P. "Changes in cortisol and testosterone levels and T/C ratio during an endurance competition and recovery." *J Sports Med Phys Fitness* 40 (2000): 139–144.

Filaire, E., Bernain, X., Sagnol, M., et al. "Preliminary results on mood state, salivary testosterone: cortisol ratio and team performance in a professional soccer team." *Eur J Appl Physiol* 86 (2001): 179–184.

Passerlergue, P., Lac, G. "Saliva cortisol, testosterone and T/C ratio variations during a wrestling competition and during the post-competitive recovery period." *Int J Sports Med* 20 (1999): 109–113.

Li, X., Michell, J., Wood, S., et al. "The effect of oestradiol and progesterone on hypoglycaemic stress-induced suppression of pulsatile luteinizing hormone release and on corticotrophin-releasing hormone mRNA expression in the rat." *J Neuroendocrinol* 15 (2003): 468–476.

Talbott, 53.

125
Weinberg and Bealer, 85.

210

126
Pendergrast, 13.

"The Women's Petition Against Coffee." Trung Nguyen, Dragon Coffee. August 1, 2010. <http://www.trung-nguyen-online.co.uk/petition.html>.

127
Moisey, L., Kacker, S., Bickerton, A., et al. "Caffeinated coffee consumption impairs blood glucose homeostasis in response to high and low glycemic index meals in healthy men." *Am J Clin Nutr* 87 (2008): 1254–61.

Petrie, H., Chown, S., Belfie, L., et al. "Caffeine ingestion increases the insulin response to an oral-glucose-tolerance test in obese men before and after weight loss." *Am J Clin Nutr* 80 (2004): 22-28.

Biaggioni, I., Davis, S. "Caffeine: A Cause of Insulin Resistance?" *Diabetes Care* 25 (2002): 399-40.

Johston, K., Clifford, M., Morgan, L. "Coffee acutely modifies gastrointestinal hormone secretion and glucose tolerance in humans: glycemic effects of cholorgenic acid and caffeine." *Am J Clin Nutr* 78 (2003): 728-33.

Kolnes, A., Ingvaldsen, A., Bolling, A., et al. "Caffeine and theophylline block insulin-stimulated glucose uptake and PKB phosphorylation in rat skeletal muscles." *Acta Physiol* 200 (2010): 65-74.

Akiba, T., Yaguchi, K., Tsutsumi, K., et al. "Inhibitory mechanism of caffeine on insulin-stimulated glucose uptake in adipose cells." *Biochem Pharmacol* 68 (2004): 1929-37.

Pizziol, A., Tikhonoff, V., Paleari, C., et al. "Effects of caffeine on glucose tolerance: a placebo-controlled study." *Eur J Clin Nutr* 52 (1998): 846–9.

Graham, T., Sathasivam, P., Rowland, M., et al. "Caffeine ingestion elevates plasma insulin response in humans during an oral glucose tolerance test." *Can J Physiol Pharmacol* 79 (2001): 559–65.

Robinson, L., Savani, S., Battram, D., et al. "Caffeine ingestion before an oral glucose tolerance test impairs blood glucose management in men with type 2 diabetes." *J Nutr* 134 (2004): 2528–33.

Lane, J., Barkauskas, C., Surwit, R., et al. "Caffeine impairs glucose metabolism in type 2 diabetes." *Diabetes Care* 27 (2004): 2047–8.

Greer, F., Hudson, R., Ross, R., et al. "Caffeine ingestion decreases glucose disposal during a hyperinsulinemic-euglycemic clamp in sedentary humans." *Diabetes* 50 (2001): 2349–54.

Lane, J., Hwang, A., Feinglos, M., et al. "Exaggeration of post-prandial hyperglycemia in patients with type 2 diabetes by administration of caffeine in coffee." *Endocr Pract* 13 (2007): 239–43.

Keijzers, G., de Galan, B., Tack, C., et al. "Caffeine can decrease insulin sensitivity in humans." *Diabetes Care* 25 (2002): 364–9.

Thong, F., Derave, W., Kiens, B., et al. "Caffeine-induced impairment of insulin action but not insulin signaling in human skeletal muscle is reduced by exercise." *Diabetes* 51 (2002): 583–90.

Thong, F., Graham, T. "Caffeine-induced impairment of glucose tolerance is abolished by beta-adrenergic receptor blockade in humans." *J Appl Physiol* 92 (2002): 2347–52.

Avogaro, A., Toffolo, G., Valerio, A., et al. "Epinephrine exerts opposite effects on peripheral glucose disposal and glucose-stimulated insulin secretion: a stable label intravenous glucose tolerance test minimal model study." *Diabetes* 45 (1996): 1373–8.

Hail, Cheryle R., Grossman, Mary Kay. *The Insulin-Resistance Diet*. New York: McGraw-Hill, 2007. 22.

128
Moisey, L., Kacker, S., Bickerton, A., et al. "Caffeinated coffee consumption impairs blood glucose homeostasis in response to high and low glycemic index meals in healthy men." *Am J Clin Nutr* 87 (2008): 1254–61.

Petrie, H., Chown, S., Belfie, L., et al. "Caffeine ingestion increases the insulin response to an oral-glucose-tolerance test in obese men before and after weight loss." *Am J Clin Nutr* 80 (2004): 22-28.

Biaggioni, I., Davis, S. "Caffeine: A Cause of Insulin Resistance?" *Diabetes Care* 25 (2002): 399-40.

Johston, K., Clifford, M., Morgan, L. "Coffee acutely modifies gastrointestinal hormone secretion and glucose tolerance in humans: glycemic effects of cholorgenic acid and caffeine." *Am J Clin Nutr* 78 (2003): 728-33.

Kolnes, A., Ingvaldsen, A., Bolling, A., et al. "Caffeine and theophylline block insulin-stimulated glucose uptake and PKB phosphorylation in rat skeletal muscles." *Acta Physiol* 200 (2010): 65-74.

Akiba, T., Yaguchi, K., Tsutsumi, K., et al. "Inhibitory mechanism of caffeine on insulin-stimulated glucose uptake in adipose cells." *Biochem Pharmacol* 68 (2004): 1929-37.

Pizziol, A., Tikhonoff, V., Paleari, C., et al. "Effects of caffeine on glucose tolerance: a placebo-controlled study." *Eur J Clin Nutr* 52 (1998): 846–9.

Graham, T., Sathasivam, P., Rowland, M., et al. "Caffeine ingestion elevates plasma insulin response in humans during an oral glucose tolerance test." *Can J Physiol Pharmacol* 79 (2001): 559–65.

Robinson, L., Savani, S., Battram, D., et al. "Caffeine ingestion before an oral glucose tolerance test impairs blood glucose management in men with type 2 diabetes." *J Nutr* 134 (2004): 2528–33.

Lane, J., Barkauskas, C., Surwit, R., et al. "Caffeine impairs glucose metabolism in type 2 diabetes." *Diabetes Care* 27 (2004): 2047–8.

Greer, F., Hudson, R., Ross, R., et al. "Caffeine ingestion decreases glucose disposal during a hyperinsulinemic-euglycemic clamp in sedentary humans." *Diabetes* 50 (2001): 2349–54.

Lane, J., Hwang, A., Feinglos, M., et al. "Exaggeration of post-prandial hyperglycemia in patients with type 2 diabetes by administration of caffeine in coffee." *Endocr Pract* 13 (2007): 239–43.

Keijzers, G., de Galan, B., Tack, C., et al. "Caffeine can decrease insulin sensitivity in humans." *Diabetes Care* 25 (2002): 364–9.

Thong, F., Derave, W., Kiens, B., et al. "Caffeine-induced impairment of insulin action but not insulin signaling in human skeletal muscle is reduced by exercise." *Diabetes* 51 (2002): 583–90.

Thong, F., Graham, T. "Caffeine-induced impairment of glucose tolerance is abolished by beta-adrenergic receptor blockade in humans." *J Appl Physiol* 92 (2002): 2347–52.

Avogaro, A., Toffolo, G., Valerio, A., et al. "Epinephrine exerts opposite effects on peripheral glucose disposal and glucose-stimulated insulin secretion: a stable label intravenous glucose tolerance test minimal model study." *Diabetes* 45 (1996): 1373–8.

Hart, Cheryle R., Grossman, Mary Kay. *The Insulin-Resistance Diet*. New York: McGraw-Hill, 2007. 22.

129
Flores-Riveros, R., McLenithan, J., Ezaki, O., et al. "Insulin down-regulates expression of the insulin-responsive glucose transporter (GLUT4) gene: effects on transcription and mRNA turnover." *Proc Natl Acad Sci* 90 (1993): 512–516.

130
Hart and Grossman, 7.

131
Unger, Jeff. "Intensive Management of Type 2 Diabetes." *Emergency Medicine*. August 1, 2010.
<http://www.emedmag.com/html/pre/fea/features/101501.asp>.

132
Chaput, J., Tremblay, A., Rimm, E., et al. "A novel interaction between dietary composition and insulin secretion:

effects on weight gain in the Quebec Family Study." *Am J Clin Nutr* 87 (2008): 303-309.

133
Chaput, J., Tremblay, A., Rimm, E., et al. "A novel inter-action between dietary composition and insulin secretion: effects on weight gain in the Quebec Family Study." *Am J Clin Nutr* 87 (2008): 303-309.

134
Moisey, L., Kacker, S., Bickerton, A., et al. "Caffeinated coffee consumption impairs blood glucose homeostasis in response to high and low glycemic index meals in healthy men." *Am J Clin Nutr* 87 (2008): 1254–61.

Petrie, H., Chown, S., Belfie, L., et al. "Caffeine ingestion increases the insulin response to an oral-glucose-tolerance test in obese men before and after weight loss." *Am J Clin Nutr* 80 (2004): 22-28.

Biaggioni, I., Davis, S. "Caffeine: A Cause of Insulin Resistance?" *Diabetes Care* 25 (2002): 399-40.

Johston, K., Clifford, M., Morgan, L. "Coffee acutely modifies gastrointestinal hormone secretion and glucose tolerance in humans: glycemic effects of cholorgenic acid and caffeine." *Am J Clin Nutr* 78 (2003): 728-33.

Kolnes, A., Ingvaldsen, A., Bolling, A., et al. "Caffeine and theophylline block insulin-stimulated glucose uptake and PKB phosphorylation in rat skeletal muscles." *Acta Physiol* 200 (2010): 65-74.

Akiba, T., Yaguchi, K., Tsutsumi, K., et al. "Inhibitory mechanism of caffeine on insulin-stimulated glucose uptake in adipose cells." *Biochem Pharmacol* 68 (2004): 1929-37.

Pizziol, A., Tikhonoff, V., Paleari, C., et al. "Effects of caffeine on glucose tolerance: a placebo-controlled study." *Eur J Clin Nutr* 52 (1998): 846–9.

Graham, T., Sathasivam, P., Rowland, M., et al. "Caffeine ingestion elevates plasma insulin response in humans during an oral glucose tolerance test." *Can J Physiol Pharmacol* 79 (2001): 559–65.

Robinson, L., Savani, S., Battram, D., et al. "Caffeine ingestion before an oral glucose tolerance test impairs blood glucose management in men with type 2 diabetes." *J Nutr* 134 (2004): 2528–33.

Lane, J., Barkauskas, C., Surwit, R., et al. "Caffeine impairs glucose metabolism in type 2 diabetes." *Diabetes Care* 27 (2004): 2047–8.

Greer, F., Hudson, R., Ross, R., et al. "Caffeine ingestion decreases glucose disposal during a hyperinsulinemic-euglycemic clamp in sedentary humans." *Diabetes* 50 (2001): 2349–54.

Lane, J., Hwang, A., Feinglos, M., et al. "Exaggeration of post-prandial hyperglycemia in patients with type 2 diabetes by administration of caffeine in coffee." *Endocr Pract* 13 (2007): 239–43.

Keijzers, G., de Galan, B., Tack, C., et al. "Caffeine can decrease insulin sensitivity in humans." *Diabetes Care* 25 (2002): 364–9.

Thong, F., Derave, W., Kiens, B., et al. "Caffeine-induced impairment of insulin action but not insulin signaling in human skeletal muscle is reduced by exercise." *Diabetes* 51 (2002): 583–90.

Thong, F., Graham, T. "Caffeine-induced impairment of glucose tolerance is abolished by beta-adrenergic receptor blockade in humans." *J Appl Physiol* 92 (2002): 2347–52.

Avogaro, A., Toffolo, G., Valerio, A., et al. "Epinephrine exerts opposite effects on peripheral glucose disposal and glucose-stimulated insulin secretion: a stable label intravenous glucose tolerance test minimal model study." *Diabetes* 45 (1996): 1373–8.

Hart, Cheryle R., Grossman, Mary Kay. *The Insulin-Resistance Diet*. New York: McGraw-Hill, 2007. 22.

135
Petrie, H., Chown, S., Belfie, L., et al. "Caffeine ingestion increases the insulin response to an oral-glucose-tolerance test in obese men before and after weight loss." *Am J Clin Nutr* 80 (2004): 22-28.

136
Björntorp, P." Neuroendocrine perturbations as a cause of insulin resistance." *Diabetes Metab Res Rev* 15 (1999): 427-41.

Björntorp, P., Rosmond, R. "Visceral obesity and diabetes." *Drugs* 58 (1999):S13-8, 75-82.

137
Boden, G., Sargrad, K., Homko, C., et al. "Effect of a low-carbohydrate diet on appetite, blood glucose levels, and insulin resistance in obese patients with type 2 diabetes." *Annals of Internal Medicine* 142 (2005): 403–411.

138
MacLean, P., Zheng, D., Jones, J., et al. "Exercise-Induced Transcription of the Muscle Glucose Transporter (GLUT 4)

Gene." *Biochemical and Biophysical Research Communications* 292 (2002): 409-414.

Thong, F., Derave, W., Kiens, B., et al. "Caffeine-induced impairment of insulin action but not insulin signaling in human skeletal muscle is reduced by exercise." *Diabetes* 51 (2002): 583–90.

Halberg, N., Henriksen, M., Söderhamn, N., et al. "Effect of intermittent fasting and refeeding on insulin action in healthy men." *J Appl Physiol* 99 (2005): 2128-2136.

Dela, F. "On the influence of physical training on glucose homeostasis." *Acta Physiol Scand Suppl* 635 (1996): 1–41.

Dela, F., Larsen, J., Mikines, K., et al. "Insulin-stimulated muscle glucose clearance in patients with NIDDM. Effects of one-legged physical training." *Diabetes* 44 (1995): 1010–1020.

Dela, F., Mikines, K., Von, L., et al. "Effect of training on insulin-mediated glucose uptake in human muscle." *Am J Physiol Endocrinol Metab* 263 (1992): E1134–E1143.

Dela, F., Ploug, T., Handberg, A., et al. "Physical training increases muscle GLUT4 protein and mRNA in patients with NIDDM." *Diabetes* 43 (1994): 862–865.

139
Thong, F., Derave, W., Kiens, B., et al. "Caffeine-induced impairment of insulin action but not insulin signaling in human skeletal muscle is reduced by exercise." *Diabetes* 51 (2002): 583–90.

140
Chiu, K., Chu, A., Go, V., et al. "Hypovitaminosis D is as-

sociated with insulin resistance and beta cell dysfunction."
Am J Clin Nutr 79 (2004): 820–825.

141
Halberg, N., Henriksen, M., Söderhamn, N., et al. "Effect
of intermittent fasting and refeeding on insulin action in
healthy men." *J Appl Physiol* 99 (2005): 2128-2136.

142
Petrie, H., Chown, S., Belfie, L., et al. "Caffeine ingestion
increases the insulin response to an oral-glucose-tolerance
test in obese men before and after weight loss." *Am J Clin
Nutr* 80 (2004): 22-28.

143
Kerr D., Sherwin R., Pavalkis F., et al. "Effect of caffeine on
the recognition of and responses to hypoglycemia in humans." *Ann Intern Med.* 119 (1993): 799-804.

Cherniske, 87.

144
Knowler, W., Barrett-Connor, E., Fowler, S., et al. "Reduction in the incidence of type 2 diabetes with lifestyle inter-
vention or metformin." *New England Journal of Medicine*
346 (2002): 393–403.

145
Newsom, S., Schenk, S., Thomas, K., et al. "Energy deficit
after exercise augments lipid mobilization but does not contribute to the exercise-induced increase in insulin sensitivity." *Journal of Applied Physiology* 108 (2010): 554–560.

146
Pendergrast, xv.

147
Cherniske, 256.

Rogers, P., Richardson, N., Elliman, N. "Overnight caffeine abstinence and negative reinforcement of preference for caffeine-containing drinks." *Psychopharmacology* 120 (1995): 457-62.

Yeomans, M., Mobini, S., Chambers, L. "Additive effects of flavour-caffeine and flavour-flavour pairings on liking for the smell and flavour of a novel drink." *Physiol Behav* 92 (2007): 831-9.

Yeomans, M., Spetch, H., Rogers, P. "Conditioned flavour preference negatively reinforced by caffeine in human volunteers." *Psychopharmacology* 137 (1998): 401-9.

Tinley, E., Durlach, P., Yeomans, M. "How habitual caffeine consumption and dose influence flavour preference conditioning with caffeine." *Physiol Behav* 82 (2004): 317-24.

Tinley, E., Yeomans, M., Durlach, P. "Caffeine reinforces flavour preference in caffeine-dependent, but not long-term withdrawn, caffeine consumers." *Psychopharmacology* 166 (2003): 416-23.

148
Herbert, Frank. *Dune*. Pennsylvania: Chilton Book Company, 1965.

149
Smith, Barry D., Tola, Kenneth. "Caffeine: Effects on Psychological Functioning and Performance." *Caffeine*. Ed. Gene A. Spiller. Florida: CRC Press, 1998.

150
Smith, Barry D., Tola, Kenneth. "Caffeine: Effects on Psy-

chological Functioning and Performance." *Caffeine.* Ed. Gene A. Spiller. Florida: CRC Press, 1998.

151
Smith, Barry D., Tola, Kenneth. "Caffeine: Effects on Psychological Functioning and Performance." *Caffeine.* Ed. Gene A. Spiller. Florida: CRC Press, 1998.

152
Smith, Barry D., Tola, Kenneth. "Caffeine: Effects on Psychological Functioning and Performance." *Caffeine.* Ed. Gene A. Spiller. Florida: CRC Press, 1998.

Strain, E., Mumford, G., Silverman, K., et al. "Caffeine dependence syndrome. Evidence from case histories and experimental evaluations." *JAMA* 272 (1994): 1043-8.

153
Smith, Barry D., Tola, Kenneth. "Caffeine: Effects on Psychological Functioning and Performance." *Caffeine.* Ed. Gene A. Spiller. Florida: CRC Press, 1998.

Silverman, K., Evans, S., Strain, E., et al. "Withdrawal syndrome after the double-blind cessation of caffeine consumption." *N Engl J Med* 327 (1992): 1109-1114.

Pendergrast, 416.

154
Hughes, J., Higgins, S., Bickel, W., et al. "Caffeine Self-administration, Withdrawal, and Adverse Effects Among Coffee Drinkers." *Arch Gen Psychiatry* 48 (1991): 611-617.

Hughes, J., Oliveto, A., Bickel, W., et al. "Caffeine self-administration and withdrawal: incidence, individual differences and interrelationships." *Drug Alcohol Depend* 32 (1993): 239-46.

Rogers, P., Martin, J., Smith, C., et al. "Absence of rein-forcing, mood and psychomotor performance effects of caffeine in habitual non-consumers of caffeine." *Psychopharmacology* 167 (2003): 54-62.

155
Heatherley, S., Hancock, K., Rogers, P. "Psychostimulant and other effects of caffeine in 9- to 11-year-old children." *J Child Psychol Psychiatry* 47 (2006): 135-42.

156
Phillips-Bute, B., Lane, J. "Caffeine withdrawal symptoms following brief caffeine deprivation." *Physiol Behav* 63 (1997): 35-9.

Rogers, P., Richardson, N., Elliman, N. "Overnight caffeine abstinence and negative reinforcement of preference for caffeine-containing drinks." *Psychopharmacology* 120 (1995): 457-62.

Hughes, J., Higgins, S., Bickel, W., et al. "Caffeine Self-administration, Withdrawal, and Adverse Effects Among Coffee Drinkers." *Arch Gen Psychiatry* 48 (1991): 611-617.

Lane, J. "Effects of brief caffeinated-beverage deprivation on mood, symptoms, and psychomotor performance." *Pharmacol Biochem Behav* 58 (1997): 203-8.

157
Strain, E., Mumford, G., Silverman, K., et al. "Caffeine dependence syndrome. Evidence from case histories and experimental evaluations." *JAMA* 272 (1994): 1043-8.

Griffiths, R., Chausmer, A. "Caffeine as a model drug of dependence: recent developments in understanding caffeine withdrawal, the caffeine dependence syndrome, and

223

caffeine negative reinforcement." *Nihon Shinkei Seishin Yakurigaku Zasshi* (Japanese Journal of Psychopharmacology) 20 (2000): 223-31.

Hughes, J., Oliveto, A., Helzer, J., et al. "Should caffeine abuse, dependence, or withdrawal be added to DSM-IV and ICD-10?" *Am J Psychiatry* 149 (1992): 33-40.

Hughes, J., Oliveto, A., Liguori, A., et al. "Endorsement of DSM-IV dependence criteria among caffeine users." *Drug Alcohol Depend* 52 (1998): 99-107.

Griffiths, R., Bigelow, G., Liebson, I. "Human coffee drinking: reinforcing and physical dependence producing effects of caffeine." *J Pharmacol Exp Ther* 239 (1986): 416-25.

158
Smith, Barry D., Tola, Kenneth. "Caffeine: Effects on Psychological Functioning and Performance." *Caffeine.* Ed. Gene A. Spiller. Florida: CRC Press, 1998.

Weinberg and Bealer, 304.

Attwood, A., Higgs, S., Terry, P. "Differential responsiveness to caffeine and perceived effects of caffeine in moderate and high regular caffeine consumers." *Psychopharmacology* 190 (2007): 469-77.

Smit, H., Blackburn, R. "Reinforcing effects of caffeine and theobromine as found in chocolate." *Psychopharmacology* 181 (2005): 101-6.

Griffiths, R., Bigelow, G., Liebson, I. "Human coffee drinking: reinforcing and physical dependence producing effects of caffeine." *J Pharmacol Exp Ther* 239 (1986): 416-25.

Griffiths, R., Bigelow, G., Liebson, I. "Reinforcing effects of caffeine in coffee and capsules." *J Exp Anal Behav* 52 (1989): 127-40.

159
"Boosting Brain Power – with chocolate." February 22, 2007. *Science Daily*. August 1, 2010. <http://www.sciencedaily.com/releases/2007/02/070221101326.htm>.

160
Weinberg and Bealer, 278.

161
Weinberg and Bealer, 278.

Bernstein, G., Carroll, M., Dean, N., et al. "Caffeine withdrawal in normal school-age children." *J Am Acad Child Adolesc Psychiatry* 37 (1998): 858-65.

Heatherley, S., Hancock, K., Rogers, P. "Psychostimulant and other effects of caffeine in 9- to 11-year-old children." *J Child Psychol Psychiatry* 47 (2006): 135-42.

Temple, J. "Caffeine use in children: what we know, what we have left to learn, and why we should worry." *Neurosci Biobehav Rev* 33 (2009): 793-806.

162
Alliance for a Healthier Generation. August 1, 2010 <http://www.healthiergeneration.org>.

"School Beverage Guidelines." *American Beverage Association*. August 1, 2010. <http://www.ameribev.org/nutrition--science/school-beverage-guidelines>.

163
Pendergrast, 280.

164
Cherniske, 291.

Lundsberg, Lisbet S. "Caffeine Consumption." *Caffeine.* Ed. Gene A. Spiller. Florida: CRC Press, 1998.

165
Stellman, S., Garfinkel, L. "Artificial sweetener use and one-year weight change among women." *Prev Med* 15 (1986): 195-202.

Yang, Qing. "Gain weight by 'going diet?' Artificial sweeteners and the neurobiology of sugar cravings." *Yale J Biol Med* 83 (2010): 101–108.

166
Davidson, T., Swithers, S. "A Pavlovian approach to the problem of obesity." *International Journal of Obesity* 28 (2004): 933–935.

Amy Patterson-Neubert. "Study: Artificial sweetener may disrupt body's ability to count calories." June 29, 2004. *Purdue News.* August 1, 2010. <http://news.uns.purdue.edu/html4ever/2004/040629.Swithers.research.html>.

167
Shapiro, A., Mu, W., Roncal, C., et al. "Fructose-induced leptin resistance exacerbates weight gain in response to subsequent high-fat feeding." *Am J Physiol* 295 (2008): R1370-5.

Teff, K., Elliott, S., Tschöp, M., et al. "Dietary Fructose Reduces Circulating Insulin and Leptin, Attenuates Postprandial Suppression of Ghrelin, and Increases Triglycerides in Women." *The Journal of Clinical Endocrinology & Metabolism* 89 (2004): 2963-2972.

Bray, G., Nielsen, S., Popkin, B. "Consumption of high-fructose corn syrup in beverages may play a role in the epidemic of obesity." *Am J Clin Nutr* 79 (2004): 537-43.

Bray, G. "Fructose: should we worry?" *Int J Obes* 32 (2008): S127-31.

168
Bray, G., Nielsen, S., Popkin, B. "Consumption of high-fructose corn syrup in beverages may play a role in the epidemic of obesity." *Am J Clin Nutr* 79 (2004): 537-43.

Ivy, J. "Glycogen resynthesis after exercise: effect of carbohydrate intake." *Int J Sports Med* 19 (1998): S142-5.

Forsythe, Cassandra. "The Evils of Fructose." *Testosterone Nation.*
August 1, 2010.
<http://www.tmuscle.com/free_online_article/sports_body_training_performance_nutrition/the_evils_of_fructose>.

Berardi, John, Andrews, Ryan. "Fructose Wars: The Nectar of the Gods or the Fast Track to Fatness?" *Testosterone Nation.* August 1, 2010.
<http://www.tmuscle.com/article/diet_and_nutrition/fructose_wars&cr=dietAndNutrition>.

Lowery, Lonnie. "Thank You for Guzzling Corn Syrup." *Testosterone Nation.* August 1, 2010.
<http://www.tmuscle.com/free_online_article/sports_body_training_performance_nutrition/thank_you_for_guzzling_corn_syrup>.

169
Elliott, S., Keim, N., Stern, J., et al. "Fructose, weight gain, and the insulin resistance syndrome." *Am J Clin Nutr* 76 (2002): 911–922.

Beck-Nielsen, H., Pedersen, O., Lindskov, H. "Impaired cellular insulin binding and insulin sensitivity induced by high-fructose feeding in normal subjects." *Am J Clin Nutr* 33 (1980): 273–278.

Gaby, A. "Adverse effects of dietary fructose." *Altern Med Rev* 10 (2005): 294-306.

Stanhope, K., Schwarz, J., Keim, N., et al. "Consuming fructose-sweetened, not glucose-sweetened, beverages increases visceral adiposity and lipids and decreases insulin sensitivity in overweight/obese humans." *J Clin Invest* 119 (2009): 1322–1334.

Parks, E., Skokan, L., Timlin, M., et al. "Dietary Sugars Stimulate Fatty Acid Synthesis in Adults." *American Society for Nutrition J. Nutr* 138 (2008): 1039-1046.

170
Tappy, L., Lê, K. "Metabolic Effects of Fructose and the Worldwide Increase in Obesity." *Physiol. Rev.* 90 (2010): 23-46.

171
Dennison, B., Rockwell, H., Baker, S. "Excess fruit juice consumption by preschool-aged children is associated with short stature and obesity." *Pediatrics* 99 (1997): 15–22.

172
Weinberg and Bealer, xiii.

173
Weinberg and Bealer, 103.

174
Weinberg and Bealer, 102.

Cherniske, 19, 257.

Pendergrast, 158, 301.

175
Acheson, K., Zahorska-Markiewicz, B., Pittett, P., et al. "Caffeine and coffee: their influence on metabolic rate and substrate utilization in normal weight and obese individuals." *Am J Clin Nutr* 33 (1980): 989-97.

Dulloo, A., Geissler, C., Horton, T., et al. "Normal caffeine consumption: influence on thermogenesis and daily energy expenditure in lean and postobese human volunteers." *Am J Clin Nutr* 49 (1989): 44-50.

Acheson, K., Gremaud, G., Meirim, I., et al. "Metabolic effects of caffeine in humans: lipid oxidation or futile cycling?" *Am J Clin Nutr* 79 (2004): 40-46.

Higgins, H., Means, J. "The effect of certain drugs on the respiratory and gaseous metabolism in normal human subjects." *J Pharmacol Exp Ther* 7 (1915): 1–9.

Dulloo, A., Geissler, C., Horton, T., et al. "Normal caffeine consumption: influence on thermogenesis and daily energy expenditure in lean and postobese human volunteers." *Am J Clin Nutr* 49 (1989): 44–50.

Astrup, A., Buemann, B., Christensen, N., et al. "The effect of ephedrine/caffeine mixtures on energy expenditure and body composition in obese women." *Metabolism* 41 (1992): 686–8.

Dulloo, A., Seydoux, J., Girardier, L. "Potentiation of the thermogenic antiobesity effects of ephedrine by dietary methylxanthines: adenosine antagonism or phosphodi-esterase inhibition?" *Metabolism* 41 (1992): 1233–41.

Dulloo, A., Miller, D. "Aspirin as a promoter of ephedrine-induced thermogenesis: potential use in the treatment of obesity." *Am J Clin Nutr* 45 (1987): 564–9.

Dulloo, A., Miller, D. "The thermogenic properties of ephedrine/methylxanthine mixtures: human studies." *Int J Obes* 10 (1986): 467–81.

Astrup, A., Toubro, S., Thorbek, G., et al. "Thermogenic synergism between ephedrine and caffeine in healthy volunteers: a double-blind, placebo-controlled study." *Metabolism* 40 (1991): 323–9.

Arciero, P., Gardner, A., Calles-Escandon, J., et al. "Effects of caffeine ingestion on NE kinetics, fat oxidation, and energy expenditure in younger and older men." *Am J Physiol* 268 (1995): E1192–8.

176
Dulloo, A., Geissler, C., Horton, T., et al. "Normal caffeine consumption: influence on thermogenesis and daily energy expenditure in lean and postobese human volunteers." *Am J Clin Nutr* 49 (1989): 44-50.

Astrup, A., Toubro, S., Cannon, S., et al. "Caffeine: a double-blind, placebo-controlled study of its thermogenic, metabolic, and cardiovascular effects in healthy volunteers." *Am J Clin Nutr* 51 (1990): 759-767.

177
Cherniske, 263-264.

Livermore, B. "Caffeine Boosts Eating Disorders." *Health.* June 1991: 16.

Castonguay, Thomas W. "Glucocorticoids as modulators in the control of feeding." *Brain Research Bulletin* 27 (1991): 423-428.

Talboll, 190.

Epel, E., Lapidus, R., McEwen, B., et al. "Stress may add bite to appetite in women: a laboratory study of stress-induced cortisol and eating behavior." *Psychoneuroendocrinology* 26 (2001): 37-49.

Newman, E., O'Connor, D., Conner, M. "Daily hassles and eating behaviour: the role of cortisol reactivity status." *Psychoneuroendocrinology* 32 (2007): 125-32.

Gluck, M. "Stress response and binge eating disorder." *Appetite* 46 (2006): 26-30.

Gluck, M., Geliebter, A., Hung, J., et al. "Cortisol, hunger, and desire to binge eat following a cold stress test in obese women with binge eating disorder." *Psychosom Med* 66 (2004): 876-81.

Dallman, M., la Fleur, S., Pecoraro, N., et al. "Minireview: Glucocorticoids—food intake, abdominal obesity, and wealthy nations in 2004." *Endocrinology* 145 (2004): 2633–2638.

Levine, M., Marcus, M. "Eating behavior following stress in women with and without bulimic symptoms." *Ann Behav Med* 19 (1997): 132–8.

231

Tataranni, P., Larson, D., Snitker, S., et al. "Effects of glucocorticoids on energy metabolism and food intake in humans." *Am J Physiol* 271 (1996): E317–25.

Cattanach, L., Malley, R., Rodin, J. "Psychologic and physiologic reactivity to stressors in eating disordered individuals." *Psychosom Med* 50 (1988): 591–9.

Lingswiler, V., Crowther, J., Stephens, M. "Emotional reactivity and eating in binge eating and obesity." *J Behav Med* 10 (1987): 287–99.

Telch, C., Agras, W. "Do emotional states influence binge eating in the obese?" *Int J Eat Disord* 20 (1996): 271–9.

Pirke, K., Platte, P., Laessle, R., et al. "The effect of a mental challenge test of plasma norepinephrine and cortisol in bulimia nervosa and in controls." *Biol Psychiatry* 32 (1992): 202–6.

178
Nørregaard, J., Jørgensen, S., Mikkelsen, K., et al. "The effect of ephedrine plus caffeine on smoking cessation and postcessation weight gain." *Clin Pharmacol Ther* 60 (1996): 679-86.

Cherniske, 55.

179
Dulloo, A., Duret, C., Rohrer, D., et al. "Efficacy of a green tea extract rich in catechin polyphenols and caffeine in increasing 24-h energy expenditure and fat oxidation in humans." *Am J Clin Nutr* 70 (1999): 1040-1045.

180
Cooper, Raymond, Likimani, Talash A., Morré, D. James,

and Morré, Dorothy M. "Catechins and Caffeine in Tea: A Review of Health Risks and Benefits." *Caffeine and Activation Theory: Effects on Health and Behavior*. Eds. Smith, Barry D., Gupta, Uma, Gupta, B.S. Florida: CRC Press, 2007.

181
Dulloo, A., Duret, C., Rohrer, D., et al. "Efficacy of a green tea extract rich in catechin polyphenols and caffeine in increasing 24-h energy expenditure and fat oxidation in humans." *Am J Clin Nutr* 70 (1999): 1040-1045.

182
Cooper, Raymond, Likimani, Talash A., Morré, D. James, and Morré, Dorothy M. "Catechins and Caffeine in Tea: A Review of Health Risks and Benefits." *Caffeine and Activation Theory: Effects on Health and Behavior*. Eds. Smith, Barry D., Gupta, Uma, Gupta, B.S. Florida: CRC Press, 2007.

183
Boyles, Salynn. "Study Casts Doubt on Weight Loss Supplements: Researchers Say 9 Dietary Supplements Are Not Effective for Cutting Weight." *WebMD*. July 12, 2010. August 1, 2010. <http://www.webmd.com/diet/news/20100712/study-casts-doubt-on-weight-loss-supplements>.

"Slimming supplements fail to produce weight loss results." *Endocrine Today*. July 15, 2010. August 1, 2010. <http://www.endocrinetoday.com/view.aspx?rid=66588>.

Zoler, Mitchel L. "Nine OTC Weight-Loss Agents Work No Better Than Placebo." July 12, 2010. August 1, 2010. <http://www.medconnect.com.au/tabid/84/ct1/c337606/Default.aspx>.

184
Waldbott, G., Burgstahler, A., McKinney, H. *Fluoridation: The Great Dilemma*. Coronado Press, 1978.

Lu, Y., Guo, W., Yang, X. "Fluoride content in tea and its relationship with tea quality." *J Agric Food Chem* 52 (2004): 4472-6.

185
Bobek, S., Kahl, S., Ewy, Z. "Effect of long-term fluoride administration on thyroid hormones level blood in rats." *Endocrinol Exp* 10 (1976): 289-95.

Wang, H., Yang, Z., Zhou, B., et al. "Fluoride-induced thyroid dysfunction in rats: roles of dietary protein and calcium level." *Toxicology and Industrial Health* 25 (2009): 49-57.

See also:
Shomon, Mary J. *The Thyroid Diet*. New York: HarperCollins, 2004;
Rosenthal, Sara M. *The Thyroid Sourcebook*. New York: McGraw-Hill, 2009.

186
Cao, J., Luo, S., Liu, J., et al. "Safety evaluation on fluoride content in black tea." *Food Chemistry* 88 (2004): 233-236.

187
Gomez, S., Weber, A., Torres, C. "Fluoride content of tea and amount ingested by children." *Odontol Chil* 37 (1989): 251-5.

188
Mercola, Joseph. "Get That Fluoride Out of Your Tea!" *Mercola.com* February 09, 2005. August 1, 2010. <http://

articles.mercola.com/sites/articles/archive/2005/02/09/
fluoride-tea.aspx>.

Hinely, P. "Greater Concentrations Of Fluoride In Tea Than
Once Thought." *Medical News TODAY*. July 15, 2010. August 1, 2010.
<http://www.medicalnewstoday.com/articles/194832.
php>.

189
Schuld, Andreas. "Green Tea, Fluoride & the Thyroid."
Parents of Fluoride Poisoned Children (PFPC). August
1, 2010. <http://www.poisonfluoride.com/pfpc/html/
green_tea____.html>.

190
Committee on Fluoride in Drinking Water, National Re-
search Council. *Fluoride in Drinking Water: A Scientific
Review of EPA's Standards*. Washington D.C.: National
Academies Press, 2006. 196-198.

191
Committee on Fluoride in Drinking Water, 218

192
Chrousos, et al., "CRH, Stress and Depression: An Etiologi-
cal Approach." Las Vegas, NV: *Conference on Cortisol and
Anti-Cortisols*, 1997.

Talbott, 104.

193
Jalali, Rehan. "Muscle Breakdown: Is Cortisol Leading You
Down the Catabolic Pathway?" *MesoRx*. August 1, 2010.
<http://www.mesomorphosis.com/articles/jalali/cortisol.
htm>.

194
Ikeda, T., Ito, Y., Murakami, I., et al. "Conversion of T4 to T3 in perfused liver of rats with carbontetrachloride-induced liver injury." *Acta Endocrinol* 112 (1986): 89-92.

Nomura, S., Pittman, C., Chambers, J., et al. "Reduced peripheral conversion of thyroxine to triiodothyronine in patients with hepatic cirrhosis." *J Clin Invest* 56 (1975): 643-652.

Sherlock, Sheila, Dooley, James S. *Diseases of the Liver and Biliary System.* Massachusetts: Blackwell, 2002. 447.

Rodes, Juan, et al. *Textbook of Hepatology: 2 Volume Set, From Basic Science to Clinical Practice.* Massachusetts: Blackwell, 2007. 1747.

195
Winter, Brian. "Seafood Contamination from Gulf Oil Disaster Could Last Years." *USA Today.* May 18, 2010. August 1, 2010.
<http://www.usatoday.com/news/nation/2010-05-18-oil-spill_N.htm>.
<http://www.organicconsumers.org/articles/article_20865.cfm>.

Oceana North America. August 1, 2010.
<http://na.oceana.org>.

"Safe Seafood Guide." *Heal The Bay.* August 1, 2010.
<http://www.healthebay.org/stayhealthy/seafoodguide/default.asp>.

196
Figueiroa, M., Vieira, C., Leite, D., et al. "Green tea polyphenols inhibit testosterone production in rat Leydig cells." *Asian J Androl* 11 (2009): 362-70.

197

Susheela, A., Jethanandani, P. "Circulating Testosterone Levels in Skeletal Fluorosis Patients." *Clinical Toxicology* 34 (1996): 183-189.

Narayana, M., Chinoy, N., "Effect of Fluoride on Rat Testicular Steroidogenesis." *Fluoride* 27 (1994): 17-12.

"The reproductive effects of fluoride intake: lowered birth rates, sperm, and testosterone are all linked to fluoride." *fluoridation.com.* August 1, 2010. <http://www.fluoridation.com/sperm.htm>.

198

Salt, Chris. *10 things you need to know about losing weight.* 2009.

199

Weaver, Jacqueline. "Much Overeating Caused By Eating Too Many Flavors All At Once." *Medical News TODAY.* January 8, 2006. August 1, 2010. <http://www.medical-newstoday.com/articles/35869.php>.

200

Smith, Barry D., Tola, Kenneth. "Caffeine: Effects on Psychological Functioning and Performance." *Caffeine.* Ed. Gene A. Spiller. Florida: CRC Press, 1998.

201

Cherniske, 8, 20.

202

Smith, Barry D., Tola, Kenneth. "Caffeine: Effects on Psychological Functioning and Performance." *Caffeine.* Ed. Gene A. Spiller. Florida: CRC Press, 1998.

203
Spiller, Monica Alton. "The Coffee Plant and Its Processing." *Caffeine.* Ed. Gene A. Spiller. Florida: CRC Press, 1998.

204
Young, Simon N. "How to increase serotonin in the human brain without drugs." *J Psychiatry Neurosci* 32 (2007): 394–399.

205
Blundell, J., King, N. "Effects of exercise on appetite control: loose coupling between energy expenditure and energy intake." *Int J Obes Relat Metab Disord* 22 (1998): S22–S29.

206
Cooper, Raymond, Likimani, Talash A., Morré, D. James, and Morré, Dorothy M. "Catechins and Caffeine in Tea: A Review of Health Risks and Benefits." *Caffeine and Activation Theory: Effects on Health and Behavior.* Eds. Smith, Barry D., Gupta, Uma, Gupta, B.S. Florida: CRC Press, 2007.

207
Rosenbaum, M., Goldsmith, R., Bloomfield, D., et al. "Low-dose leptin reverses skeletal muscle, autonomic, and neuroendocrine adaptations to maintenance of reduced weight." *J Clin Invest* 115 (2005): 3579–3586.

Hill, J. "Understanding and Addressing the Epidemic of Obesity: An Energy Balance Perspective." *Endocrine Reviews* 27 (2006): 750-761.

Brown, W., Williams, L., Ford, J., et al. "Identifying the energy gap: magnitude and determinants of 5-year weight gain in midage women." *Obes Res* 13 (2005): 1431–1441.

208
Weinberg and Bealer, 93.

209
Weinberg and Bealer, 104.

210
Weinberg and Bealer, 126.

211
Pendergrast, 16.

212
Weinberg and Bealer, 291.

213
Weinberg and Bealer, 197.

214
Weinberg and Bealer, 160, 183.

Pendergrast, 300.

215
Weinberg and Bealer, 14.

216
Pendergrast, 420.

217
Jeffery, Robert W., Harnack, Lisa J. "Evidence Implicating Eating as a Primary Driver for the Obesity Epidemic." *Diabetes* 56 (2007): 2673-2676.

Flegal, K., Kuczmarski, R., Johnson, C. "Overweight and obesity in the United States: prevalence and trends." *Int J Obes* 22 (1998): 39–47.

Ogden, C., Carroll, M., Curtin, L., et al. "Prevalence of overweight and obesity in the United States, 1999–2004." *J Am Med Assoc* 295 (2006): 1549–1555.

Ogden, C., Flegal, K., Carroll, M., et al. "Prevalence and trends in overweight among US children and adolescents, 1999–2000." *J Am Med Assoc* 288 (2002): 1728–1732.

218
Hill, J. "Understanding and Addressing the Epidemic of Obesity: An Energy Balance Perspective." *Endocrine Reviews* 27 (2006): 750-761.

Bray, G., Nielsen, S., Popkin, B. "Consumption of high-fructose corn syrup in beverages may play a role in the epidemic of obesity." *Am J Clin Nutr* 79 (2004): 537-43.

Hill, J., Peters, J. "Environmental contributions to the obesity epidemic." *Science* 280 (1998): 1371–4.

Hill, J., Wyatt, H., Reed, G., et al. "Obesity and the environment: Where do we go from here?" *Science* 299 (2003): 853–855.

Hill, J., Wyatt, H., Peters, J. "Modifying the environment to reverse obesity. In: Goehl TJ, ed. Essays on the future of environmental health research." *Environmental Health Perspectives* 113 (2005): 108–115.

219
Levine, J. "Obesity: Mission Possible." *Diabetes* 56 (2007): 2653-2654.

220
Jeffery, Robert W., Harnack, Lisa J. "Evidence Implicating Eating as a Primary Driver for the Obesity Epidemic." *Diabetes* 56 (2007): 2673-2676.

Shah, M., Jeffery, R. "Is obesity due to overeating and inactivity, or to a defective metabolic rate: a review." *Ann Behav Med* 13 (1991): 73-81.

Costanza, M., Beer-Borst, S., Morabia, A. "Achieving energy balance at the population level through increases in physical activity." *Am J Public Health* 97 (2007): 520–525.

Utter, J., Neumark-Sztainer, D., Jeffery, R. et al. "Couch potatoes or french fries: are sedentary behaviors associated with body mass index, physical activity, and dietary behaviors among adolescents?" *J Am Diet Assoc* 103 (2003): 1298–1305.

Hamilton, M., Hamilton, D., Zderic, T. "Role of low energy expenditure and sitting in obesity, metabolic syndrome, type 2 diabetes, and cardiovascular disease." *Diabetes* 56 (2007): 2655–2667.

221
Jeffery, Robert W., Harnack, Lisa J. "Evidence Implicating Eating as a Primary Driver for the Obesity Epidemic." *Diabetes* 56 (2007): 2673-2676.

222
Levine, J. "Obesity: Mission Possible." *Diabetes* 56 (2007): 2653-2654.

INDEX

Made in the USA
Monee, IL
23 February 2020